SOLVING THE BIG, FAT PUZZLE

How to create a sustainable solution

that works for YOU!

Disclaimer

This book is meant to serve as a collection of strategies based on the collective personal experiences of the author. Your actual results may vary. The reading of this book does in no way guarantee your results will mirror those of the author.

The author of this book has made all reasonable efforts to provide current and accurate information for the readers of this book. Whether because of the progression of the Internet, or the unforeseen changes in company policy and editorial submission guidelines, what is stated as fact at the time of this writing may become outdated or inapplicable later. The author and her associates will not be held liable for any unintentional errors or omissions that may be found.

The author and publisher are providing this book and its contents on an "as is" basis and make no representations or warranties of any kind with respect to this book or its contents. The author and publisher disclaim all such representations and warranties, including for example warranties of merchantability and healthcare for a particular purpose. In addition, the author and publisher do not represent or warrant that the information accessible via this book is accurate, complete or current.

The statements made about products and services have not been evaluated by the U.S. Food and Drug Administration. They are not intended to diagnose, treat, cure, or prevent any condition or disease. Please consult with your own physician or healthcare specialist regarding the suggestions and recommendations made in this book.

Except as specifically stated in this book, neither the author or publisher, nor any authors, contributors, or other representatives will be liable for damages arising out of or in connection with the use of this book. This is a comprehensive limitation of liability that applies to all damages of any kind, including (without limitation) compensatory; direct, indirect or consequential damages; loss of data, income or profit; loss of or damage to property and claims of third parties.

You understand that this book is not intended as a substitute for consultation with a licensed healthcare practitioner, such as your physician. Before you begin any healthcare program, or change your lifestyle in any way, you should consult your physician or another licensed healthcare practitioner to ensure that you are in good health and that the examples contained in this book will not harm you.

This book provides content related to physical and/or mental health issues. As such, use of this book implies your acceptance of this disclaimer.

FORWARD

There are very few moments in your life when you meet someone and instantly know that they are uniquely authentic. Johnette van Eeden is such a person. I have never met anyone with such innate drive and perseverance. Many people want to have their own venture; however, few are willing to do the work required to make their vision into reality. Johnette has the natural talent to take an idea and see it through to completion, with the final outcome far exceeding the original goal.

Needing to lose a few pounds myself, I was a curious observer as she successfully progressed towards her goal, without the rollercoaster "gain and lose" that you normally see when people attempt to lose weight. I have been impressed not only in her achievement, but more so that she has been so successful in keeping it off! I have already implemented some of the changes she outlines here and look forward to learning more details as she shares more of her journey in this book.

Johnette's drive to do whatever it takes also carries over into her personal life. I would probably not be alive today if not for her. When my wife voiced concerns about me to Johnette, she immediately jumped into action and was able to schedule a vascular screening within a few hours. When the results showed a carotid blockage, she personally spoke with the Radiologist, and my personal Cardiologist, to share the findings. She then drove me to the emergency room herself, coordinating with my wife where to meet, and even had her husband collect & look after my dog. Had she not stayed to help argue my case with the ER doctor I might not be here today, since he wanted to send me home without treatment. I am pleased to report I have fully recovered from a successful endarterectomy, a surgery in my neck to remove the plaque blockage. My vascular surgeon told me I narrowly avoided having a catastrophic stroke!

Johnette has repeatedly shown that when she says she is going to do something that it WILL happen. Her personal accountability and integrity are beyond question. I have mentored scores of entrepreneurs during my life, but I can honestly say she is my favorite student. The world needs more entrepreneurs as dedicated to success, both personally and professionally, as her! I am fortunate to call her friend.

Jay D Rodgers, Serial entrepreneur, Mentor, & Biz Owner's Ed Founder

ENDORSEMENTS

Johnette has it figured out – you first gotta know how it really works and once you do - it's up to you! I encourage you to read this book to learn from her years of solid research and proving those learnings on herself. ~ **Tony Jeary - The RESULTS Guy™**

Johnette has written a heart-felt, easy to follow book for those struggling to meet personal weight and health goals. In my practice, I see clients who struggle with controlling their blood sugar, blood pressure, and the weight gain from insulin resistance. Working with patients to control their food intake and deal with the emotions involved is not an easy task for any practitioner. Johnette provides a guide that is easy to read and easy for anyone, regardless of income, to put into practice. A must read for anyone looking for a lifestyle, not a fad diet, to put into practice for weight loss and add more life to their years. ~ **Kenneth Wightman, MSc, ND**

This book is such an amazing resource about the reality of obesity and how to actually tackle weight loss effectively. Over the years since I met Johnette I've learned she is an excellent source for honest information, especially when it comes to personal wellness. Witnessing her transformation has been great motivation not to mention proof it really works and is sustainable! ~ **Jillian House, Texas**

I have known Johnette and worked with her for quite a number of years. During this time, I have seen her in action, putting into practice the current understanding of functions involved in good health. She's helped quite a number of people including myself to become healthier. Her book is a must-read and is a recap of her journey and discoveries. I highly recommend that anyone interested in improving their health read this book. She has helped me immensely in my own journey to Better Health. ~ **B Koehn, Ft. Worth**

Johnette is an ambitious student of anything she puts her sights on. She is passionate about weight loss and the health benefits of a strong weight loss program that is scientifically based. She is living proof of the fruits of her research on the subject, as well as putting her knowledge to use personally and professionally. Our practice has utilized the research and knowledge Johnette has done to benefit our patients in their weight loss journey, which in turn has had a positive impact on their overall health. ~ **Kayleigh King, APRN, FNP**

Johnette only writes about topics for which she has applied 'a personal test' with corresponding success! My dear friend of many years offers here a welcome addition to this critically important subject. ~ **Roger Price, BA, M.Ed., CTVI**

Somewhere in Johnette's life someone told her she could be or do anything she put her mind to...and she has. It is inspiring to see her take a topic as complex as weight loss and break it down into small, understandable pieces that we can all learn from. Her perseverance is encouraging to watch as she continues to soar. ~ **Tamara G**

Johnette's weight loss journey has been such an inspiration to me. Her knowledge of nutrition and intermittent fasting have helped me become more aware of what I am putting into my body, encouraging me to be healthier. She really is a walking testimony of what she speaks. It's refreshing to see a book not about some fad diet, but other topics as well, like your mindset, and how even small changes there help enable you to make healthier choices. ~ **D.B., Texas**

I have known Johnette for over 25 years. I've seen her excel at everything she gets her hands on (from computer programming to medical screening). She will pick up an interest and break it down until it makes sense to her. And

then she will graciously share this newfound knowledge to anyone who is willing to listen. There is no better person to look into obesity and weight loss than Johnette, her research as well as her own experiences with the topic will be an eye-opening revelation to many. ~ **Caro B, Atlanta**

I have looked on with admiration at the progress of Johnette's transformation as she steadily lost her weight. Sustained weight loss is a seemingly out-of-reach goal for most of us, but I am not surprised that Johnette has succeeded. She is determined, astute, and practices what she preaches. Her honesty and compassion make her the ideal person to offer advice to others attempting to achieve improved wellness.
~ **Tina Maree, Australia**

I have known Johnette van Eeden for over 15 years. She has always been dedicated to "Wellness" and has been very involved in helping others by offering various blood tests, ultrasound screenings, and other options to help people with early detection of disease processes and disease prevention. Given her personal success, I think you will find her book about her own weight loss journey very informative.
~ **Sadie P, RN, BSN**

I have had the pleasure of working with Star Wellness for several years to provide shot clinics for our employees. Johnette has always been a pleasure to work with and thinks about what we need and how they can assist with promoting the health and wellness of our employees. She is both professional and personable, putting customer service first and providing a valuable service to our community. Fort Worth is lucky to have her! ~ **Sarah King, PHR, M.S., Health and Wellbeing Manager**

Johnette van Eeden and Star Wellness are a great asset to the Grandview School District. She and her staff are always available in any situation. We have had fewer absences of staff due to their onsite flu shot clinics for our employees and children. This saves on our substitute budget throughout our district, and we are getting a $1000 bonus check for it! Our employees love the lipotropic and B12 shots, which have helped numerous employees lose weight and feel better. Last year at this time, I was critically ill with an arthritis issue. I was able to regain my strength twice as fast by taking advantage of their vitamin B12 shots! Johnette is always available for any questions or concerns I may have; I've never been told she is too busy for my call. At GVISD, we all love her and Star Wellness! ~ **Lisa Davis, RN**

I have known Johnette van Eeden for three years in a professional relationship. We have worked together to understand the hidden world around us, and I have seen her put in the time and effort to take her knowledge to another level. Johnette is a tenacious student of all things regarding health. I have witnessed this journey of weight release that she has traveled and I am impressed. I am looking forward to applying the things she has learned to my own life to release excess weight I have maintained from my years as a chef. ~ **Tom Heintz, Holistic Healing Practitioner**

Johnette van Eeden is an outstanding entrepreneur. She believes in applying the highest standards for anything to which she attaches her name. She is knowledge, reputable, heath conscious, honest and very personable. When something needs doing, she will start, attacking with purpose, and won't stop until it is completed, no matter how long or how difficult. Her weight loss is inspiring - she is truly an awesome lady! ~ **Bettye Rodgers, RN**

PREFACE

In 2000, the World Health Organization predicted that diabetes would grow at an alarming rate, reaching 366 million worldwide by the year 2030.

They missed the mark by grossly UNDERestimating. By 2015 the number of people with diabetes was already 415 million, up from 171 million, in only 15 years!

Today, 1 out of every 11 adults worldwide is already diabetic. The updated figures from 2015 now predict 642 million diabetics by 2040.

This is truly staggering. How can this be? How could their estimate be so far off the actual diabetes numbers? The answer: obesity. And, mostly due to dietary habits and lifestyle choices.

Type 2 Diabetes & Obesity, now collectively called "Diabesity", will soon be the number one killer of the human race – WORLDWIDE. This means that for the first time in history, the next generation is projected to have a shorter life-expectancy. We are literally eating ourselves to an early grave by becoming obese younger.

The economic ramifications of this global epidemic are staggering as well – over $2 Trillion in 2014 for healthcare costs related to obesity. Indirect costs from reduced productivity and/or inability to work add even more. Two-thirds of filed bankruptcy are due to medical issues. Allowed to continue, treatment costs alone will lead to catastrophic economic consequences worldwide.

We have made incredible advances in medicine yet obesity and diabetes rates continue to rise. We have to reverse this trend, and quickly, in order to survive.

The medical community has proven to be ineffective in regards to sustainable weight loss. The promoted mantra is still "eat less, move more", with many even going further, telling patients to eat 5-6 "small" meals per day. In most cases this advice is completely counterproductive!

I firmly believe that most people want to have a healthy diet and lifestyle, but simply do not know what to do or eat. We are bombarded daily with mixed and often conflicting information. Unfortunately, this is not limited to only the

U.S., but has become an epidemic for any country that has embraced the Western diet (i.e. "processed foods").

The time has come for everyone to accept personal responsibility and take control of their health. This begins with our lifestyle choices, including our diet. Is it easy? No, but that does not mean that it can't be done.

Thousands of people, including myself, have successfully lost weight, stopped the progression of chronic diseases, and even reversed their diabetes.

I am confident that you can too!

Table of Contents

CHAPTER 1

INTRODUCTION

You've been lied to.

The simple truth is that we all have been lied to by the so called "experts" and medical community when it comes to weight loss. The common thought and recommended mantra for weight loss over the past few decades (more than 30 years!) has been "eat less, move more"; count your calories and simply burn more calories than you consume. Just increase your exercise to burn additional calories. What a load of garbage!

Losing weight is not that simple. Has this plan worked for you or anyone you know long term? Have you dieted before and lost weight only to gain it all back once you stop? I have, and chances are you have too.

Eat less, move more simply does not work! It has been an epic fail with a 99% long-term failure rate, yet most physicians still recommend this as their primary protocol, then blame the patient when it fails, claiming they must not be following the recommended guidelines.

Worse, it is discouraging and demoralizing to anyone who is overweight because it simplifies the issue too far, making it sound like the problem is just them.

Obesity is much more complicated than this catch phrase and there are numerous pieces to the puzzle other than just diet and exercise. Everyone is unique; there is no one size fits all formula. What works for Mike may not be effective for Mary.

All calories are not created equal either! If they were, eating 100 calories of cookie and 100 calories of celery would have the same impact on the body. They simply do not and you instinctively understand this already.

According to the National Institutes of Health, obesity and overweight together are the second leading cause of preventable death in the United States, behind tobacco.

An estimated 300,000 deaths per year are due to the obesity epidemic in the U.S. and the estimated cost of obesity in the U.S. is $147-210 billion annually. Medical costs for an obese patient presenting to the emergency room with chest pains are 41% higher than a normal weight person.

Obesity is also the leading cause of Type II diabetes, the 7th leading cause of death in the U.S. and responsible for 10% of health care dollars. A diabetic employee generates an estimated $8,000 more in health care expenditures to the company health plan each year than a non-diabetic employee. Diabetes is also the leading cause of blindness in working-age adults, affecting more than half of the 18 million people over the age of 18 with diabetes in the U.S., according to the NIH.

And, it's not limited to just the United States. The World Health Organization reports that obesity has nearly tripled worldwide since 1975. Even more alarming is the fact that over 380 million **CHILDREN** were overweight or obese in 2016!

When I turned 50, I realized that I wasn't simply overweight anymore, I was actually classified as obese. I had been eating what I considered a healthy diet, but was still gaining 2-5 pounds per year. The extra pounds I had put on would inevitably lead to chronic disease. I was 45 pounds overweight and headed towards metabolic syndrome, insulin resistance, and developing type II diabetes.

Knowing that the body functions best at an optimal weight, I decided to get to the root of the issue and determined to figure my weight loss dilemma out for good. This book is to share my journey and what I learned through this process with you. I have shared the information contained within this book with numerous friends and others who have also had similar success with losing weight and keeping it off.

While the steps are fairly simple, it is not easy. But, as **Paulo Coelho** so aptly stated, *"There are some things in life that are worth fighting for to the end. You are worth it."*

You and your health, my precious reader, are so worth it! Besides, if you don't take care of your health and your body, where else are you gonna live?

By the time you finish reading this book you will learn:

- The different way your body gets fuel for energy.
- How to get your body to burn your stored fat for its energy needs.
- How to read and understand nutrition labels on products.
- How to plan, shop, and prep your food.

- Detailed steps to begin losing the stubborn weight you've been trying to lose for so long.

- What to do to keep that weight off.

Let me tell you more about how I got to this point.

CHAPTER-2

MY PERSONAL JOURNEY

As a child, I was raised in a small Texas town in a relatively rural community. My grandparents lived next door, and my grandfather was a truck farmer who raised tomatoes, squash, and cucumbers. One of our "neighbors" (meaning within 5 miles) was a dairy farmer. In the summer I was ready to be in the fields to start work by 6:00 am. In the Texas heat we had a small window in the mornings to harvest for the day, before the temperature became too hot. We were outside in the sunshine and got Vitamin D every day.

We also had a family garden and raised much of our own food. My grandmother and mother would also "can" fresh vegetables from our garden during the summer so we would have them to eat during the winter. We even made our own pickles and salsa.

We rarely went out to eat. My mother, with our help, would make dinner from scratch each evening. Going to McDonald's or out for ice cream was a special treat. We had three meals a day and were rarely allowed snacks. Our drink choices were water, iced tea without sugar, or milk. Sodas were a very rare privilege.

The children played outside during the day and we played in the dirt (gasp!) and got dirty! So much so that there would be a noticeable amount of sand in the bathtub each evening after all four of us were bathed and the water was drained! We rode our bicycles, ran, and played hide-and-seek or tag a lot.

During my middle school years my small town went through a construction boom and a huge influx of new families moved into the area. Farmland was sold and neighborhoods were constructed. Our rural community became more urban. Restaurants and fast food places quickly followed. We even had a 7-11 convenience store built only one mile away, so we could now walk down the road to get a Slurpee!

Fast forward and take a look at childhood today. Certainly, the childhood of my own children, who were even raised in the same city, was remarkably different!

Rarely does a family have a garden where they grow most of their own food. It is almost unheard of that people "can" their own food for the winter. Eating out is the norm; the family dinner is rare, or even non-existent, for many children. Soda is the primary beverage consumed daily, and sometimes the only beverage. Many children never even drink water during the course of a day. Is it any wonder why we have a worldwide epidemic of obesity?

Kids rarely play outdoors, and if they do, they do not actually get dirty. Studies have found that exposure to dirt has many health benefits. Did you know that dirt has been shown to help boost the immune system and functions as a natural anti-depressant? Do not be afraid to play in the dirt!

In 2002, I began research and work in the Wellness Industry as a result of some personal health issues within my immediate family. My own research helped me see what supplements I needed to consume to optimize our health, given the issues and concerns of my family.

While there were a lot of supplements claiming to cure you of anything that ails you, no one was doing any testing to see if any of them actually worked! I started my medical screening company as a way to test blood levels and determine if supplements were actually doing what they claimed. Fifteen years later my company, Star Wellness®, is considered one of the top onsite biometric screening companies in the United States.

While my company was growing, my waistline was growing as well. I was eating what I considered a healthy diet and taking supplements, yet I continued to gain 2-4 pounds a year. For the most part I chalked this up to aging and going through menopause. I told myself that I needed some fat reserves in case I got ill during my senior years, right? Wrong. I had slowly become clinically obese.

My fasting glucose was going up as well. My father had already been diagnosed as a Type II diabetic, was obese, and had already had bypass surgery. I knew that I was becoming metabolic resistant, and quickly on my way to developing diabetes myself, if I did not get the weight off. I was approached about an opportunity to open a new medical clinic, with providers that would offer medically supervised weight loss. Someone recommended that we purchase an InBody scale which provides comprehensive Body Composition Analysis so we ordered the 570 model.

We set up the scale and I got on to see how it worked. I tend to have small arms and legs because I carry most of my weight in my midsection, however I was shocked to see how high my visceral fat level was!

What is visceral fat? It's the fat that is stored around your internal organs in the abdominal cavity. Visceral fat is what makes you out of breath as you bend over to tie your shoes because it presses on your lungs. Visceral fat is also linked to increased risk for several long-term and life-threatening diseases. Visceral fat is dangerous and I knew I had to reduce this number if I wanted to stop my progression towards becoming insulin resistant and diabetic myself.

But what could I do that would work? I had already tried Atkins, Paleo, Keto, and other "fad" diets. While I would lose some weight initially, I would always gain it back since this way of eating was not really sustainable.

I'm a native Texan, and we tend to be somewhat stubborn. Once we set our mind on something it's difficult to get us off that course. I was determined to figure out why I was not having much success in losing weight. **This book is to share this awakening and life-changing journey with you.**

While attending a Flourish retreat for women, hosted by my friend Cyndee Jardieu, I heard a woman named Amber speak about intuitive eating. What she said resonated with me so I set up a call with her to learn more. With her help I learned how to slow down and listen to what my body was telling me it needed prior to eating. I learned to make peace with food and honor my hunger. She taught me to have compassion for myself whenever I "failed" and helped me to see my blind spots and limiting beliefs surrounding food. We also talked about how many times people eat for emotional reasons and not actual hunger.

This process awakened a desire in me to know more, which led me to read The Emotion Code, by Dr. Bradley Nelson. This book helped me to see that I, like everyone, had situations and circumstances that happened during my lifetime, that resulted in emotions becoming "trapped". We often refer to this as "emotional baggage". While still skeptical, I found a certified emotional code practitioner in my area and set an appointment.

From my first meeting with Tom Heintz I was completely hooked! What a powerful experience for me and wonderfully fulfilling career path for him. What could be more rewarding than helping others to identify and release their emotional baggage? I was blown away. He knew nothing about me, yet he was able to simply muscle test and tell me about an injury I had to my left elbow, including the year of the injury - 1982! How was he able to be so accurate with information that happened years ago by simply muscle testing?

This was my first true exposure to energy work and how everything is interconnected. I referred my husband and several friends to Tom, all of whom had similar experiences.

Around this time as well I was told about a documentary series that was available called *"iThrive! Rising from the depths of Diabetes & Obesity"*. My husband and I watched some of this and soaked in what the experts being interviewed were saying. During episode 8 of this wonderful series, there is an interview with Dr. Jason Fung, a nephrologist at the University of Toronto in Canada. He has a very successful diabetes reversal program, with thousands of patients successfully reversing their diabetes!

Remember, doctors tell you that diabetes is a chronic disease, meaning you will have it for the rest of your life. The normal train of thought in the medical community is that you cannot reverse diabetes, yet Dr. Fung PROVES it is actually reversable, and, even better, fairly easy to reverse! I intuitively knew this was the path I must travel to get to my ultimate destination and optimal weight.

There are other things I learned along the way as well, such as the necessity of your mindset, using meditation and affirmations for success in weight loss, and the importance of sleep & hydration. We will cover all of this and more in the next few chapters.

Today my BMI is at a normal level – I am no longer obese. I successfully lost 40 pounds over a seven-month period, but more importantly, have been successful at keeping it off. I was even able to wear the perfect dress at my daughter's wedding! My bloodwork looks great, I lowered my A1c from 6.1% (prediabetes level) to 5.3% (normal)! I now have more energy and feel better than I have in years.

I have shared my path with others and they have had success as well. It's an exciting journey, and the path is unique for each person. As you can already see, there are multiple pieces to the puzzle, but I'm confident that by the end of this book you will be able to figure out how to put your individual puzzle pieces together.

Ready to get started?

CHAPTER 3

EVERYTHING IS ENERGY

"If you want to know the secrets of the universe, think in terms of energy, frequency and vibration."
~ Nikola Tesla

For some of you, this area may be challenging to your belief systems. Many, and probably most, of us were brought up to believe in science from a Newtonian point of view. That is to say that if something is to be true you must be able to measure and "prove" it to be true. This way of thinking has actually shaped our way of thinking for centuries.

Quantum physics however proves that everything in the universe is made up of energy and that solid matter really does not exist. How is this possible?

Everything is made up of atoms. But what are atoms made from? If you zoom in on one, you will see that they have three subatomic particles: electrons, neutrons, and protons. The neutrons and protons are clustered in the middle with the electrons zooming around this center so rapidly they cannot really be tracked. So, in essence, if atoms are really energy, and everything is made of atoms, then everything is made up of energy.

This is an oversimplification of a complex topic, but this has actually been proven multiple times. Now, take a moment and try to wrap your brain around this fact. Take your time. Reread the previous paragraph if necessary....

Once you understand and comprehend that we are all made up of energy, I want you to also realize that you radiate a **unique energy signature** into the universe. No one else will ever have the same energy signature that you do! It is also interesting to note that the largest electromagnetic field emanating from your body is generated by the heart, not the brain. This energy field can even be measured for up to 8 feet away from the body!

There is a fascinating video called "*Mysteries of the Heart*" by the Institute of Heartmath on YouTube I would encourage you to watch to learn more.

Where this topic gets really interesting is when you take it to the next step and see that this energy signature can truly be altered by consciousness. Quantum entanglement proves that once particles interact with one another, they remain "entangled", even when separated by a large distance. This means that if you alter a measurable outcome to one set of particles, the equal and opposite affect will happen on any other set of entangled particles **simultaneously**. This proves that everything is made up of energy and it is all interconnected!

Confused? I was at first as well. But when you really stop and think about it for a moment it makes perfect sense.

Bring to mind someone you know who is positive, funny, and generally upbeat. They come into the room and everyone's mood improves. You have a yearning to be close to them because you immediately are drawn to their positive energy. And, if you were feeling low, just being around them helps to lift you up as well.

Now think about someone who is usually negative, depressed, or angry. It's the exact opposite. You immediately dread being around them because you do not want to be sucked into their negative energy. Just being in their presence drains energy from you and makes you feel worse.

How many times before have you been thinking about someone and the phone will ring with that person on the other end? This is also the result of interconnected energy.

Personally, my goal is to give as much positive energy into the world as I can, and I now understand that just by consciously shifting my emotions I can also shift my unique energy signature to help me accomplish this goal.

Heart-mind congruence

Have you ever wanted to achieve something, yet you end up doing something else and self-sabotaging your efforts? It has happened to everyone at one point or another and it happens in dieting all the time. You wake up and say to yourself – "I'm going to do this today! I'm going to follow my plan, no cheating".

Then the day starts and life gets in the way. It turns out that there is a birthday party celebration at work, complete with birthday cake, and you only had salad for lunch so you start thinking, "I've been good today, I'll get a small piece of cake, but just have a bite and not eat the whole thing." Next you rationalize this by telling yourself "besides, if I don't have cake and participate in the celebration, everyone will think I'm not a team player".

By making the decision about being a team player, you have just justified the decision to eat cake in your head. So, you go ahead and accept a piece of cake with everyone else. Before you know it, you have eaten the entire piece and then find yourself saying yes to a second!

Nothing changed in these few moments except the conversation in your head where you convinced yourself, while denying your instinct, in order to justify the decision. This process is called self-deception.

Having your heart and mind in congruence helps in making these decisions without the self-deception. It is difficult to stop self-sabotage when your mind is telling you to decide in one direction, while your heart is saying to go the other. Congruence simply means that your heart and mind are in agreement so there is no rationalization to justify, the decision is automatic.

Anytime you make a change to your normal way of doing things, your subconscious will become alarmed and send you conflicting signals, preferring to remain in the more comfortable state of "this is the way we have always done this". In order to make a change successfully, you need to consciously rewire your thinking. This is possible, it just takes a little effort.

Have you ever known someone who fully embodied their personal core values? This is a person who does not hesitate when making a decision. They seem to instinctively know which way to decide so they do not have to consciously think about the decision, they can just act. There is no effort involved, it's an automatic reaction. That is what it means to practice heart-mind congruence.

People are attracted to others who are congruent. We often recognize this without realization, and refer to this as charisma. The most successful people in the world, also some of the most congruent, are naturally congruent. They instinctively "practice what they preach" and others recognize this in their authenticity. They wholly believe in what they say and do, so they are by default more genuine and believable. Others WANT to be around them.

This is the type of person I strive to be more like each day. My goal is to be authentic, living my life on purpose, and surrounded by others who feel the same.

Now that you understand the importance of heart-mind congruence, how do you put it into practice? How can you achieve this for yourself? You have to get out of your own head and listen to your heart, then simply connect the two.

For me it took some time to sit and think about where I was, where I wanted to be, and what it would take to make that journey. I also found small amounts of focused meditation helped, but we will discuss that more in a later chapter.

Think about and concentrate on your ideal image, on where you ultimately want to be. What does it feel like? What are you wearing? What does it look like? Who are you with? Sense the temperature of the room, the smells in the air, and hear the background noises around you. Engage as many senses as possible in your scenario.

Doing this simple exercise really does create an emotional connection between your heart and mind, to the desired outcome of your goal, that you can refer back to time and time again. Some people even take this a step further and create a vision board, where they take that imagined outcome and make it visual, posting images that help to visually represent their goals. They place this in an area they can easily see each day to help them remain on track.

Whenever you have doubts or questions simply take a moment to make this connection again in your mind. The more you do this the easier it becomes to imagine and see clearly each time. This simple mind exercise helps to reinforce your WHY for the changes you are making on your journey to optimal health and wellness; and makes all the challenging decisions you need to make on the way far easier.

The great news about this technique is that it works for any topic or goal you may set for yourself, not only dieting and weight loss.

CHAPTER 4

HOW THE BODY GETS ENERGY

Now that we understand that everything is made up of energy, we need to shift to thinking about the energy sources our body uses for fuel. Metabolism is the method by which the body breaks down fuel sources, converting them into energy.

In order to successfully achieve weight loss, you must get your body to use the fat it has stored for energy. Sounds easy, right? But if that is all there is to it, then why is it so hard? To answer this question, we first need to have a basic understanding of how the body gets fuel.

There are only two fuel sources available in the body: glucose or stored fat. However, the body can only use **one fuel source at a time!** My goal is to help you understand the difference between the two and how to get you out of the glucose state more efficiently so you can burn your stored fat for fuel. While I am not a doctor and this is a gross simplification of the process, you can find more information online or on our website – www.BigFATPuzzle.com.

To your body, glucose is easier to use and a more readily available fuel source. When your body has glucose available it remains in a "fat-storing" state. It will stay in this state as long as it can, placing any excess glucose into long-term storage, inside the fat cells. While you are in the fat storing state, the body will continue to store away any excess, resulting in weight gain. This is the default state that most people stay in almost all the time.

Carbohydrates, such as starches and sugars, are converted by the body into glucose. The glycemic index is a value given to different foods to show how quickly it will raise blood glucose levels.

Think about the standard American diet (the SAD diet). What do most people, and especially children, eat for breakfast? Usually it is cereal, pancakes, toast, bagels, or donuts. All of these are simple carbohydrates that are quickly converted to glucose by the body!

After a few hours, or even less time since simple carbs digest faster than whole foods, lunch usually consists of a burger and fries or sandwich and chips – a very heavy simple carb load again. And, what are most people drinking? The majority of people will have a soda, which is full of sugar! Most people will drink at least a 20-ounce serving (or more). I mean, you have to get your money's worth by opting for the free refill, right?

Take a guess regarding how much sugar is in a single 20-ounce bottle of soda. The answer may shock you – 60 grams of sugar!

I realize this does not mean much to most people so I would like to explain 60 grams of sugar a bit further. A packet of sugar, like one you would add to your cup of coffee, is typically 4 grams. That means that when you consume a 20-ounce soda, and for many people this is multiple times a day, you are actually eating 15 of those sugar packets!

Would you put 15 packets of sugar into anything you normally drink? No! Yet, many Americans routinely drink sodas without giving it a second thought. And we wonder why we keep gaining weight?!

To get your body into a fat burning state, where it uses stored fat for fuel, you must first deplete the body of all available glucose and eat fewer calories than you burn. But this is not as easy as it sounds either because, of course, everyone's metabolism is different. What effectively works for Linda may have the opposite effect for Mary. We have all seen this happen time and time again, which is why "dieting" does not work!

By restricting the total amount of simple carbohydrates you consume, you will deplete the body of available glucose faster, and your body will convert to the opposite process, called the "fat burning" state. Increasing the amount of time between meals also helps to deplete the glucose reserves faster.

This fat burning state is where everyone wants to be so they will burn stored fat and lose weight, however we have a very difficult time getting here. Generally, this is because, as we have shown above, we are constantly replenishing the glucose available to the body by the kind of foods we consume.

When you are in the fat burning state, fat cells are pulled from their long-term storage inside your fat cells and consumed by the body for energy. This process is called ketosis and is the basis for several "low carb" diets that are popular today. We will cover more about these later.

Simple carbs, like bread or candy, are made from refined, processed carbohydrates (white flour and sugar), and have a high glycemic index. This simply means they will digest and convert to glucose in the body much faster than a complex carb, like vegetables, fruits, or whole grains. Surprisingly, some of them even convert to sugar in the body faster than sugar itself!

This explains why simple carbohydrates are the carbs to avoid. The easy way to remember a large portion of this group is to think white: white flour, white sugar, white rice, potatoes, and bread. All of these are simple carbs that quickly convert to sugar for your body to store as fat!

Alternatively, complex carbohydrates, such as vegetables, are generally lower in sugar and high in fiber, causing them to breakdown slower in the body and taking two to three hours to digest. The easiest way to start learning the difference is to review a glycemic chart for foods. On the chart, each item listed is assigned a value of 0-100, with 100 representing pure glucose. Values are assigned based on the blood glucose level two hours after ingesting the item. The general guideline is that carbohydrates with a glycemic index value of 55 or less are preferred, although recent reports say less than 45 is even better.

Another way to measure how quickly a food will spike blood glucose level is glycemic load, which measures the amount of carbohydrates in a single serving of a particular food item. A glycemic load of ten or less is considered a good food choice, a score of ten to twenty will have a moderate impact on your blood sugar level, and a food falling into the over twenty category will cause a spike in your blood glucose level. Understanding both glycemic index and glycemic load will give you a more complete picture of how particular foods will affect your blood sugar level.

There are numerous charts and guidelines available online showing the glycemic index and glycemic load of various foods. I encourage you to find one that is easy for you to understand and use. Print out a copy that you can refer to as an aid in making better, and healthier, food choices.

There is a very good reason for why your mother always said to "eat your veggies!".

CHAPTER 5

THE IMPORTANCE OF
BASELINE TESTING

As the old adage goes, "you can't change what you don't measure". It is important to get baseline information prior to starting any new program and to help identify any potential underlying health conditions. For this reason, we always recommend a routine check-up with your personal physician prior to starting any type of new weight loss program.

While I am not a doctor, so I do not diagnose or prescribe, here are the baseline testing our clinic sees most frequently recommended by physicians for individuals looking to start a weight loss program:

Basic Labs & measurements for everyone:

- Height/Weight/BMI

- Waist, hip, bust, & chest circumference

- Body Fat Percentage

- Blood Pressure

- **Comprehensive Metabolic Panel (CMP)** – a 14 panel test of electrolyte levels, as well as kidney and liver functions, glucose, calcium, & proteins.

- **Complete Blood Count (CBC)** – a panel to measure levels of the cells that make up your blood to detect a wide range of issues, including infection, anemia, & leukemia.

- **Fasting Lipid Panel** – a panel to measure the components of cholesterol: Total cholesterol, LDL, HDL, VLDL, & triglycerides.

- **Thyroid Stimulating Hormone (TSH)** – a standard thyroid function test.

- **Hemoglobin A1c with eAG** – a test to assess glucose control and/or diabetes.

- **Vitamin D, 25-Hydroxy** – a test to measure the blood serum level of vitamin D, important for immune health. It is estimated that 75% of Americans are deficient without supplementation. Recent studies indicate that a level of 80-100 ng/mL is optimal.

Additionally:

Basic physical fitness assessment (with modification if necessary):

- Stretch & reach

- Number of Jumping Jacks in 30 seconds

- Number of Squats in 30 seconds

- Number of Sit-ups in 30 seconds

For new patients, our medical providers also like to see:

- **Magnesium, RBC (not serum level)** – a measurement of the magnesium level in the red blood cells.

- **Zinc** – a measurement of zinc levels in the blood. Zinc is a trace mineral found in all body tissues.

- **Vitamin B12 & Folate** – a measurement of B12 & folate levels, both are needed by the body to function normally.

- **Ferritin** – a measurement of the ferritin protein in the blood to see the level of iron stored in the body.

- **Free T3 (FT3)** – the form of thyroid called triiodothyronine that is unbound and available for use in the body.

- **Free T4 (FT4)** – the form of thyroid called thyroxine; used to further evaluate thyroid function.

- **Reverse T3 (RT3)** – the inactive form of triiodothyronine; used to further evaluate thyroid function.

"In my 28 years of medical practice and teaching, I have found that nutrient testing is critical for health optimization. Zinc is an important mediator of healing and inflammation reduction, acts as an aromatase blocker, and promotes good estrogens. According to some authorities zinc deficiency in the United States is regularly overlooked. Indications of zinc deficiency include loss of appetite, hair loss, poor wound healing, and impaired immune function. Low levels have also been linked with depression and dementia.

RBC magnesium is another frequently overlooked test and suboptimal levels are common. Magnesium is an important cofactor in over 300 body reactions and has roles in carbohydrate and lipid metabolism. Low magnesium can contribute to nerve irritability spasm of any type of muscle including coronary (it is a treatment for life-threatening cardiac arrhythmias), skeletal muscle (goes hand-in-hand with calcium and muscle metabolism as well as bone, and preventing osteoporosis), intestinal, and urinary smooth muscle; therefore, it aids in digestion, bowel regulation, and blood pressure regulation.

Serum magnesium is a poor measure to follow since it is not an accurate reflection of total body supply. RBC magnesium follows the body supply more linearly and is a more accurate reflection of tissue adequacy.

I have found that the middle of normal range should be used as the cutoff for optimization of both zinc and RBC magnesium." ~ **Randall Hayes, D.O.**

Baseline testing is absolutely essential prior to starting any new program, both for ruling out underlying conditions and measuring effectiveness throughout the program. Additional information is also available on our website.

CHAPTER 6

WHAT DO I EAT?

"Eat food, not too much. Mostly plants."
– Michael Pollan

The above quote by Michael Pollan probably makes more sense to me than anything else I've seen or read in regards to eating for optimal health and wellness. Time and time again studies have shown that a whole-foods, plant-based (WFPB) diet is the optimal diet for humans. In fact, when all popular diets were compared in a scientific study by Yale University, real food was the winner, not only in meeting nutritional needs, but in reduction of cancer and heart disease as well.

What you eat really does matter!! As Hippocrates said – *"Let food be thy medicine"*!

According to research published in the *Journal of the American Medical Association*, modifiable behavioral risk factors are the leading cause of death in the U. S., with diet listed as one of the primary lifestyle factors blamed for half of all deaths, second only to tobacco use. Researchers also estimate that poor diet and lack of physical activity will soon overtake tobacco as the leading cause of death!

Eat like your life depends on it – because it ultimately does! My dear friend Cyndee likes to ask herself before she eats – "Is this going to heal my body, or hurt my body?", and then decides accordingly.

The next question everyone asks is "what does whole foods mean"? I like to think of it this way: if it did not grow out of the ground or have a mother, you should not eat it. Being minimally processed is the key; if it has been heavily processed, you should avoid eating.

This means highly refined grain products like white flour, white sugar, or white rice are to be avoided. You want the foods you consume to be as they are in nature, not highly processed.

With only a few exceptions, if a food product will not spoil or go bad within a few days it is not a whole food. Generally speaking, prepared foods that will not spoil, or have an extended shelf life, are not good for your health or body.

Adopting a WFPB mindset simply means returning to a simplified way of eating, arguably a more natural way of eating, that includes whole foods and spices for flavoring.

Another benefit from following a more WFPB way of eating is that it is environmentally friendly. Animal farms require lots of water, land, and energy, producing a considerable amount of waste. The animal eats plants to convert them into muscle tissue. A single cow will eat up to 28 pounds of hay per day and needs about an acre and a half of land! Once the animal gets to the acceptable size and weight, they must be transported for sale. From there they are usually transported again for slaughter and packaging. Then the packaged items require being transported again (this time with refrigeration) for distribution to the store for you to purchase.

The whole-foods, plant-based diet is also one of the easiest to follow. You do not have to necessarily count carbs or calories, simply eat from a wide range of whole foods, including vegetables, fruits, legumes, seeds, nuts, & whole grains.

People tell me all the time that they cannot eat this way because they do not like to eat vegetables. I always challenge them to roast their vegetables in the oven. While microwaved or steamed cauliflower or Brussel sprouts are often flavorless, when roasted they are absolutely delicious! Plus, you can eat all of them you want. My husband and I will frequently eat an entire head of roasted cauliflower during one meal – it really is that delicious!

A WFPB diet avoids using animal products, dairy, sugar, and added fats as much as possible. Am I saying that you are never allowed to have these again? No, not at all. It is virtually impossible to avoid these all together, especially in certain social settings. Moderation and being sensible is really the key. I personally try not to consume meat in my home, but will eat it when dining out with others if no other item on the menu appeals to me. If I feel like a steak, I will have a steak and not feel any guilt.

The necessity of eliminating sugar

"I'm serious when I say that evidence is mounting that too much added sugar could lead to true addiction." – **Alan Greene, MD**

Remembering that healthy weight loss depends on depleting our glucose reserves so that the body will make the switch to burning fat for energy, we want to eat accordingly. The most efficient way to accomplish this is to eat foods that are low in sugar, with a low glycemic index, and avoid foods that are high in sugar or have a high glycemic index.

Most importantly, sugar is off limits. It is the primary source of glucose and is highly addictive, more so than even cocaine! It is also hidden in many various forms and under different names, in almost all processed foods.

Common FDA recognized "hidden" names for sugar:

Agave Nectar/Syrup	Diastatic malt	Maltodextrin
Beet sugar	Ethyl maltol	Maltose
Blackstrap molasses	Evaporated cane juice	Maple syrup
Brown rice syrup	Florida crystals	Molasses
Brown sugar	Fructose	Muscovado sugar
Cane juice	Fruit juice	Nectars
Cane sugar	Galactose	Panela sugar
Caramel	Glucose	Piloncilo sugar
Carob syrup	Glucose syrup	Powdered sugar
Castor sugar	Golden sugar	Raw sugar
Coconut sugar	Golden syrup	Refiner's syrup
Confectioner's sugar	Grape sugar	Rice syrup
Corn syrup	High-Fructose Corn Syrup (HFCS)	Sorghum syrup
Corn syrup solids	Honey	Sucanat

Crystalline fructose	Icing sugar	Sucrose
Date sugar	Invert sugar	Sugar (granulated)
Demerara sugar	Jaggery sugar	Syrup
Dextrin	Lactose	Treacle
Dextrose	Malt syrup	Turbinado sugar

Your body will not like being deprived of processed sugar. In the beginning, you may even feel bad for a few days as you go through the sugar withdrawal process. It is common to notice cravings, have low energy, or headaches. These are simply withdrawal symptoms because your body is so used to having an unlimited supply of glucose available. The carb addiction will usually take about four days to break, so hang in there! You CAN do this.

Foods to consume:

- Non-starchy vegetables (raw or cooked), unlimited quantity

- Whole foods (single ingredient; will spoil)

- Low-glycemic fresh fruits (berries, small quantities)

- Nuts & seeds, moderate (small handful)

- All spices

Foods to eat in moderation:

- Starchy vegetables (peas, potatoes, sweet potatoes, etc.)

- Whole fruits (not juiced or dried, watch glycemic levels)

- Avocados & Coconut (due to high fat content)

- Beans & Legumes

- Gluten-free grains

- Dairy, limited

- Small portions of lean protein (rarely, no larger than your palm)

Foods to avoid:

- All processed food

- Food that does not spoil (i.e. Twinkies, Oreos, etc.)

- High sugar foods (candy, cakes, cookies, etc.)

- Dried fruits

- Corn

- Refined flours & sugars

- Sugary beverages (soda, fruit juice, sports drinks, etc.)

- Alcohol

Avoid snacking as it will also cause a spike in glucose levels and promote fat storage. Late night eating impairs fat burning while you sleep, increases inflammation and insulin levels, and interferes with healing and repair of the body.

Ideally you should only eat 2-3 meals a day, spaced at least 4 hours apart with no snacking. To avoid getting famished gradually increase spacing between meals to allow your body time to adjust. Again, any withdrawal symptoms you may experience (being jittery, irritable, and feeling weak) generally will subside after about four days.

All eating should be complete at least three hours before you go to bed, with optimal bedtime being between ten and eleven o'clock in the evening. The longer you have between dinner and breakfast the next morning the longer your 'fast', which allows your body additional time to pull from its stored fat reserves for energy.

Again, you CAN do this!! When you get frustrated, just remember the only thing you really have to lose is weight!

CHAPTER 7

VITAMINS ARE IMPORTANT

"There are pleasures in eating good foods and a varied diet.
That's a reason to not just live on pills."
– Bruce Ames, Ph.D., biochemist, age 90

First, I want to clarify that if you are following a whole-foods, plant-based diet and eating a wide variety of vegetables, nuts, and fruit, you are ahead of the game in meeting many of your nutritional needs with diet alone. Optimizing vitamin & mineral levels is advantageous in helping you on the journey to your weight goal.

However, even with a WFPB diet, you still need to supplement. According to a study from the *International Journal of Obesity*, people who take a multivitamin while continuing to eat their normal diets, lost an average of about three and a half pounds over six months. Those who took a placebo lost nothing.

While there is no magic pill for optimal health, you do want to ensure that your body is getting the essential vitamins and minerals it needs. Most diets for weight loss involve some type of caloric restriction. Taking good quality supplements each day ensures that your body is still properly supported during this period. This not only prevents nutritional deficiencies, but also reduces disease risk and helps support athletic performance as well.

Recent research reports that most people are deficient in many key nutrients and states that taking vitamins and supplements to optimize these levels could "*add a few years to everyone's life*".

When your body is deficient in necessary nutrients, it will pull what it needs from anywhere it can find in the body, which can compromise your long-term health. An example would be the body taking magnesium stored inside cells to protect against DNA damage, for the purpose of relieving a muscle cramp. Sure, the muscle cramp will resolve, but at a potentially high cost. It really is short-term gain with long-term consequences.

Do not sacrifice your longevity because you do not want to take a vitamin!

My family has taken vitamins & supplements for years. I'm even so geeky that I have a spreadsheet for everything we take with ingredients listed to ensure the combined levels are correct. People sometimes think we are crazy but we hardly ever get sick and avoid taking prescription medications.

I take my supplements first thing in the morning to prepare my body for the day. For some vitamins and minerals, more is not better. Fat-soluble vitamins, like vitamins A, D, E, and K, are stored by the body for later usage. Taking too much can cause excess accumulation and, in some cases, damage. Water-soluble vitamins, such as most B vitamins and C, are filtered out by the kidneys and removed from the body via urination. This is why your urine may change color shortly after taking them.

Remember how we discussed the importance of baseline blood testing earlier? Testing helps to identify deficiencies and dosage for certain vitamins and minerals. We always advise that you speak with your personal physician prior to taking new supplements, especially if you are on any prescription medications. Certain supplements can interfere with medications or may need to be taken separately.

Amazingly though, most medical schools teach very little on nutrition, vitamins, and supplements. According to **David Eisenberg, an adjunct associate professor of nutrition at Harvard T.H. Chan School of Public Health**, speaking to *PBS NewsHour* - *"Today, most medical schools in the United States teach less than 25 hours of nutrition over four years. The fact that less than 20 percent of medical schools have a single required course in nutrition, it's a scandal. It's outrageous. It's obscene"*.

Moreover, most of the training provided to doctors during medical school focuses on identification of vitamin deficiencies, such as scurvy (vitamin C) and beriberi (vitamin B1), which are not as prevalent in current times. Even though current guideline recommendations list nutrition as a primary course of care, do not be surprised if your doctor is hesitant or tells you vitamins are useless. It might be that he simply does not have adequate training in nutrition to answer your questions.

Vitamin D, magnesium RBC, zinc, vitamin B12, folate, & zinc are all included on the list of 41 nutrients medically proven necessary to help you live longer, published in October 2018 by the Proceedings of the National Academy of Sciences. It is amazing how much better you will feel if you just optimize these few!

"Vitamin D is regarded as one of the most important nutrients for our health. It regulates more than 2,000 of the 30,000 human genes and plays a significant role in immune function and physical performance. Vitamin D also helps the body absorb calcium, subsequently helping build bones and keep them strong and healthy. Many people hear "Vitamin D" and think of exposure to the sun. This is an accurate correlation, as vitamin D is produced in your skin in response to sunlight. However, if you live in non-equatorial latitudes, the sun may not be strong enough to produce vitamin D for about half of the year, making supplementation necessary. In fact, as many as one billion people worldwide are estimated to be vitamin D-deficient. Sustained levels of vitamin D deficiency can result in brittle bones, bone pain, as well as muscle pain and weakness." ~ **Kenneth A. Wightman, ND, MS**

Our Provider Recommended Daily Supplements:

1. A good quality multivitamin - a good quality brand will contain a balanced formula of bioavailable vitamins and minerals that are often deficient in the modern diet. The formula should include a balanced blend of essential antioxidant vitamins A, C, and E, and a complex of B vitamins, along with calcium, magnesium, and zinc for optimal bone and metabolic health. Avoid hard pressed tablets and opt for capsules instead for better absorption. Better quality capsules will require 4 or more per day.

2. Omega 3 (Fish Oil) –at least 2000-3000 mg of EPA and DHA combined each day for optimal results.

3. Vitamin D – our clinic recommends Douglas Labs D-Sorb, a small, easy to swallow capsule containing 12,500 IU of vitamin D3 in a patented, naturally self-assembling nano-colloid system for enhanced absorption. More than seventy-five percent of Americans are deficient in Vitamin D and it is virtually impossible to get to the new recommended optional range of 80-100 ng/dL without supplementation.

4. Vitamin K - is primarily known for its role in blood clotting. It also helps with calcium absorption in the bones & teeth, while helping to reduce accumulation of calcium in soft tissues. It is important to take Vitamin K and Vitamin D together. Again, consult with your physician prior to taking, especially if you are on a blood thinner for any reason.

5. Digestive Enzymes - active whole-food enzymes and supporting cofactors that are frequently deficient in most diets to support the body's production of enzymes critical for digestion of food and healthy function. Recommended dosage of 1-2 with your supplements and at the beginning of meals for additional digestive support.

6. Probiotics - live microorganisms that encourage friendly bacterial growth. Our providers recommend a probiotic that provides a delivery system designed to help protect the sensitive probiotic cultures from stomach acid to ensure delivery into the gut.

Additional supplements, if recommended:

Time Release Iron (only if needed from blood test results) – Time Release Iron tablets are specially designed to provide iron over a six to eight-hour period. Carbonyl iron is well-tolerated, easily absorbed, and has a low toxicity.

Zinc (if blood testing results are low)

Magnesium (if RBC blood testing results are low)

DigestZen Digestive Blend Softgels - While their primary purpose is to support proper digestion and gastrointestinal tract health, these softgels also ease feelings of queasiness, including discomfort caused by motion or activity. Also available in a chewable calcium carbonate tablet form.

And, of course, any other supplement recommended by your personal healthcare provider.

CHAPTER 8

UNDERSTANDING NUTRITION LABELS

"To eat is a necessity, but to eat intelligently is an art." ~
La Rochefoucauld

Learning to read and understand the nutritional label on food products will help you to make healthier dietary decisions. Below is a glossary of key terms included in the Nutrition Facts label found on consumable foods. When comparing choices between similar products, the information on the label can aid you in selecting a healthier option.

The label is divided into four sections. The top section shows the serving size and servings per container. It can be quite a shock for some people to learn that what they typically eat as a serving is actually multiple servings!

Below this, in the second section, is calories per serving. If the package is two servings and you eat the entire package, you will need to multiply by two (or more). The general guideline for calories is 100 calories per serving is considered moderate, 40 is low, and 400 calories or more is high.

The next section lists key nutrients that you may want to limit, such as fat, cholesterol, sodium, sugar, and protein, along with the percentage of daily value (%DV) each serving contains of these nutrients. Remember, not all fats are necessarily bad. You want to limit saturated fats and avoid trans-fat. Total sugars will include both natural and added sugars.

The fourth section lists nutrients that you want to ensure you get enough of each day from your diet: vitamin A, vitamin C, calcium, iron, & dietary fiber. Use this section to help limit or increase these nutrients as needed.

At the bottom of the nutrition label you will find a footnote stating "% DVs are based on a 2,000-calorie diet.", which is mandatory for all food labels. Additional information may also be available if the package is not too small. This area is where you will find what percentage of the recommended daily value is contained in a serving, based on a 2,000 or 2,500 calorie per day diet.

Glossary of Key Nutrition Label Terms

Calcium: a mineral that builds and maintains strong bones. Calcium helps prevent osteoporosis.

Calories: the energy provided by food/nutrients. On the label, calories shown are for **one serving** only.

Nutrition Facts

Serving Size 1/4 Cup (113g)
Servings Per Container 8

Amount Per Serving

Calories 100	Calories from Fat 20

	% Daily Value*
Total Fat 2g	3%
Saturated Fat 1.5g	7%
Trans Fat 0g	
Cholesterol 10mg	3%
Sodium 460mg	19%
Total Carbohydrate 4g	1%
Dietary Fiber 0g	0%
Sugars 4g	
Protein 16g	

Vitamin A 0%	•	Vitamin C 0%
Calcium 8%	•	Iron 0%

* Percent Daily Values are based on a 2,000 calorie diet.

Calories from Fat: Fat calories shown on the label are for **one serving** only.

Cholesterol: a necessary nutrient that is carried in the bloodstream. LDL cholesterol is considered "bad", while HDL cholesterol is considered "good."

Daily Value: the amount of certain nutrients that most people need to consume each day.

Nutrient: an ingredient in a food that provides nourishment or nutritional benefit.

Nutrition Facts Label: the black-and-white box found on food and beverage packages.

Percent Daily Value (%DV): the percentage of a nutrient found in one serving of food, based on the established standard of 2000 calories per day.

Saturated Fat: a type of fat that is solid at room temperature. Saturated fat is usually animal-based (meat and dairy), and is associated with certain health risks.

Serving Size: how many servings are in the package. All of the nutrition information on the label is based upon one serving of the food. If the serving per container is 2, then a serving size is ½ of the container; if you eat the entire thing you must double all the information on the label because you are really eating two servings.

Sodium: dietary salt that is important in the diet. However, too much sodium can lead to high blood pressure and risk of heart disease.

Total Fat: the total contact per serving of combined fats that provide energy to the body. Some types of fat are healthier than others.

Trans Fat: a type of fat that is created when liquid fat is turned into solid fat during manufacturing. Trans fat has no daily value, and should be replaced with unsaturated fat in your diet whenever possible.

Unsaturated Fat: a type of fat that is liquid at room temperature; can be plant-based or animal-based. These are usually "good fats".

Take your vitamins and supplements! Your body will actually crave certain foods when it is low on certain vitamins and minerals. Salt cravings are often due to calcium deficiency and craving chocolate has been linked to magnesium deficiency.

CHAPTER 9

KETO AND THE PROTEIN MYTH

"We've never treated a single patient with protein deficiency; yet the majority of patients we see are suffering from heart disease, diabetes, and other chronic illnesses directly resulting from trying to get enough protein."
~ **Dr. Alana Pulde and Dr. Matthew Lederman**

Most of the information regarding high-fat, low carb diets that we have been told for the past thirty years is simply not true. Ever since the Atkins diet came onto the scene in the late 1980's there has been a continuous low-carb diet craze, with a "new" style of high-fat, low-carb, moderate (or high) protein diet becoming popular every few months.

According to Wikipedia, at the height of the Atkins diet popularity in 2003-2004, one in eleven adults in North America was following a low carb diet. Currently, we have Paleo and Keto as being the most popular. The premise of these high-fat, low-carb diets is the same as our goal - starve the body of carbs and lower glucose levels by reducing the amount of sugar consumed, to achieve ketosis, thereby getting the body to burn stored fat for energy.

My husband was a believer in the keto diet and had some success so I decided to give it a try as well. According to my ketone blood testing levels, I was successful at getting into a higher ketosis state than he was, but I ended up with gout and kidney stones as well. Not good. I also did not like having to consume additional fat and protein in order to maintain the ridiculous levels that they encourage.

Recent studies show that yes, high-fat, low-carb diets can be effective, especially short-term for initial weight loss, however the dietary restrictions required to maintain the diet are unrealistic, with a high failure rate.

Also, for most people, once carbohydrates are introduced back into the diet, the weight is gained back, often with additional pounds being added as well. We have all seen individuals who have successfully lost weight following this style of diet, but have not been able to maintain the weight loss long-term.

Plus, we know intuitively that eating all the bacon and pork rinds you want, while not being allowed to have any fruit, and even certain vegetables, cannot be good for the body. Recent medical studies indicate that following these types of diets can even be dangerous.

I have a good friend who was a big proponent of the Keto diet and initially lost some weight following the diet off and on for a couple years. He would add butter and coconut oil to his coffee in the morning and intentionally consume additional fat with meals to stay in ketosis.

His wife mentioned to me one day that she was concerned about him and some issues she had noticed recently. I suggested they have his carotid arteries scanned for blockage as his symptoms sounded like he might be experiencing "mini-strokes", or TIAs (Transient Ischemic Attacks).

As a nurse, she agreed and he consented to have the ultrasound screening. He had a blockage of over 80% on the left side, and was 50% occluded on the right as well! We immediately took him to the emergency room where, after several hours, they performed an angiogram to confirm the findings. He had to undergo a carotid endarterectomy, surgery to remove the plaque from his carotid artery, and has now recovered.

He was very fortunate that this was caught prior to having a full-blown stroke, or "brain attack", considering stroke is the leading cause of adult disability. An ischemic stroke is caused by a blockage in the arteries leading to the brain, from the formation of plaque or a blood clot.

Unfortunately, his way of eating was keeping his triglycerides level high, which studies have shown to be associated with the formation of plaque and ischemic strokes. Yes, I do know that the Keto diet can be effective at rapid weight loss for some people, and following this diet can be successful for children with epilepsy, but we still do not completely understand why this works.

The dirty secret that Keto proponents do not tell you is that the benefits of the ketogenic diet decrease over time and it actually causes an increased risk of non-alcoholic fatty liver disease, arterial stiffness (from plaque formation), and cardiovascular risk. Muscle loss is also a known side effect with the ketogenic diet.

The whole foods, plant-based diet we discussed earlier is a far better and safer way of eating to effectively burn stored fat.

The Protein Myth

Protein is not only good for muscle mass, but also for staying satiated and boosting metabolism. However, it is a widely accepted myth in our culture today that extra protein, specifically animal proteins, is REQUIRED for optimal health. This is especially pervasive with athletes who are told that without copious amounts of protein each day their athletic performance will suffer.

This unfounded myth is commonly perpetuated by large animal agriculture interests that are very well funded and effective at convincing us that we absolutely NEED their products.

We certainly need protein in our diets. However, you ARE able to get all of your protein needs via plant-based sources. In fact, almost all plant-based food contains protein. The USDA Food Composition Database reports that a 1 cup serving of broccoli has 3.71g of protein, pinto beans (3/4 cup) have 19.44g, and 1 cup of spinach has 3.99g of protein.

Additionally, diets high in plant protein are also linked to many health benefits including lower risk of heart disease, reduction in diabetes risk, and lower risk of weight gain. So, when you eat your veggies you get protein, fiber, plenty of other nutrients, and health benefits as well!

There are numerous professional athletes who have come forward recently testifying that converting to a plant-based diet has actually IMPROVED their athletic performance. In addition to better performance, they also report improved mental clarity and generally feel better overall.

Think of the numerous animal species that thrive on a plant-based diet. Do you think elephants, cows, or gorillas worry about getting enough protein? No! Yet these animals build considerable muscle mass from eating plants.

Animals convert plants to muscle tissue more easily than humans because of the amino acids that their bodies naturally produce. This is another reason why meat is promoted as necessary for consumption. It can provide many essential amino acids, "essential" meaning they must be obtained through the diet; they are not naturally produced by our bodies.

How can we ensure we get the necessary amount of essential, and non-essential, amino acids when following a WFPB diet? By eating a varied diet that includes not only vegetables and fruit, but also nuts, legumes and whole grains. And, do not forget to take your daily supplements!

Your body does not need you to overload it with protein to flourish or burn stored fat. Study after study has conclusively proven that the most effective and sustainable diet for humans is a whole food, plant-based diet. Rest in the assurance that you can get enough protein just by eating a variety of plant-based foods.

CHAPTER 10

PORTION CONTROL & CHEWING

*"A tiny change today brings a dramatically different tomorrow." ~ **Richard Bach***

Portion control is a topic that immediately scares people. We tend to think that in order to successfully lose weight we are going to have to starve ourselves. This is simply not true. Portion control does involve some discipline and self-control; however, it is fairly easy to implement once you understand a few tips and guidelines.

Many diets have failed or been undermined by our tendency to have "just one more bite." We also tend to eat multiple servings without even realizing what we are doing. No matter what type of diet you are on, identifying the correct portion size allows you to know exactly how many, or how much, calories, carbs, sodium, and fat you are consuming. It is a cornerstone to building good eating habits and increases your chance of successfully losing weight and keeping it off.

One tip that you frequently hear whenever you try a new diet is to use smaller plates to help with portion control. In America, most meals we are served in an average restaurant are enough to feed two adults. In fact, my husband and I frequently share an entrée when dining out. I also regularly divide my meal in halves when it arrives at the table and only eat half, taking the remainder home with me to enjoy at the next meal or the following day.

A second tip that I implemented early on was to slow down at meal time and intentionally chew my food longer. My personal mantra became "eat less, chew longer!". I even wrote this in large letters on the white board in my office to continually remind myself.

Chewing more has additional benefits beyond just slowing down your meal consumption. It also increases the amount of saliva and digestive juices you produce and ingest, thereby further aiding digestion.

Consciously paying attention as you eat will help you to slow down, chew longer, and enjoy your food more. We are told as children to hurry up and clean our plates. This is ingrained in many of us from childhood and a false belief that is difficult to overcome. Listen to me here – **It is perfectly OK to not eat everything on your plate!**

Slow down and enjoy your meal, savor each bite, and fellowship with those around you. We do not have to be in such a hurry to eat everything on our plate as quickly as possible. As my good friend Rick Hopper, the ReadeRest inventor and SharkTank superstar says: *"I enjoy my food much more in my mouth than I do in my stomach, so chew longer!"*.

Obviously, chewing longer makes your food particles smaller so that they are more easily digested. I know it is not a topic people like to talk about, but you should be having multiple bowel movements per day, without straining. Many people I speak with do not, and struggle to have at least one per day!

Constipation is an issue that can be eased by better chewing habits. If constipation is a problem for you, examine the amount of water and fiber you are consuming to see if either, or both, are lacking. You should speak with your personal physician if it continues more than a few days to rule out any underlying issues.

Slowing down when you eat will automatically help you to consume less as well. Did you know that once your stomach is "full" it actually takes about 20 minutes before your brain receives and acknowledges the "full" signal?

Think of a time at the end of a meal when you were completely miserable, wondering how you possibly ate so much. You think to yourself, "Why do I feel so overfull? I wasn't even this full when I stopped eating!". The answer is that you ate too fast and overfilled your stomach prior to your brain getting the signal to STOP eating! You continued eating beyond the full state. If you are not consciously aware of your eating, you can easily continue to eat and then suffer from that overfull feeling that we all have experienced.

Instead of immediately going back for a second serving during meals, wait and give your body time (10-15 minutes) to start digesting what you have already consumed. Usually, this will allow your brain to get the "full" message and the feeling of needing more will subside.

Using a scale to weigh out portions will also help you to learn correct portion size, especially in the beginning stages. It is very easy to eat more than a single serving without even realizing. I recommend that you store food items in single portion sizes so that you are not tempted to eat beyond the single serving. This also has the advantage of convenience since you do not have to think about how much of an item to take, you can just grab the single serving and enjoy.

Another side benefit of portion control is cost savings. It will actually save you money since you are consuming less! Using the practice of consciously controlling the serving sizes you consume is an effective and budget friendly way to lose weight.

Controlling portion size is relatively easy once you learn the basics and get the hang of it.

TIPS FOR CONTROLLING PORTION SIZE

At home:

- Use smaller dishes at meals.

- Serve food in single portion servings; do not go back for seconds.

- Store any leftovers in separate, single-serving amounts. Consider freezing the portions you likely will not eat for a while.

- Never eat out of the bag or carton!

- Don't keep platters of food on the table; you are more likely to "pick" at it or have a second serving without realizing it.

At restaurants:

- Ask for half or smaller portions.

- When your meal is served, immediately divide out the portion size to eat, setting the rest aside.

- Ask for a takeout container and box the remainder of your plate right away to reduce temptation.

At supermarket:

- Completely avoid the snack food aisles; sticking to the outside perimeters of the store where the whole foods are typically located.

- Make a shopping list prior to going to the store and stick to the list.

- Do not go to the store when you are hungry as you will be tempted to purchase more. Going to the store shortly after a meal, when you are already satiated, will help you to avoid impulse purchasing.

While on your personal journey to achieve optimal health and wellness, the practice of portion control is vital for a sustainable outcome. It may feel difficult at first, but like any new habit it will become second nature over time. You will start to automatically recognize when you need to stop eating and begin to give yourself permission to quit, even before your plate is empty.

CHAPTER 11

FASTING FOR HEALTH

"To eat when you are sick, is to feed your illness."
~ Hippocrates

"The best of all medicines is resting and fasting."
~ Benjamin Franklin

Fasting, in my personal experience, is by far the most effective, efficient, and neglected weight loss tool available. Fasting is a centuries-old practice of consciously not eating for a period of time, used across almost all cultures and religions for healing, cleansing, and purification. Fasting can also be very effective in helping you get past a plateau in your efforts; however, it is often underutilized, or not used at all.

Contrary to popular belief and misinformation, fasting is not bad for you, unless you are already underweight. We all instinctively know this. When you are sick, you do not feel like eating – it is the last thing you want to do. This is because your body knows it takes energy to digest any food you ingest. Your body would rather use that energy to heal.

Fasting has stood the test of time and has been utilized and recommended for centuries by many influential people. Also, it's FREE, so it actually SAVES you money, since you simply are not consuming anything during your fasting periods!

Fasting should always be done safely. This is especially important if you are on medication, are diabetic, have gout, liver, kidney, or heart disease. Long-term fasting (more than 3 days) should always be medically supervised to ensure safety. When practiced correctly and SAFELY, fasting can be far more effective than ANYTHING the medical community has to offer. Fasting is not recommended for children, during pregnancy, or for women who are nursing.

You should never feel bad when fasting. Most people report they actually feel better, have more energy, and are able to better focus. If you start to feel bad while fasting you should stop, break your fast, and have some broth or just eat a meal.

Think of the word "breakfast". When you look closely at the word you can see that it literally means to break your fast. You automatically fast overnight while you are sleeping. If you are one of the few people who get up and eat in the middle of the night, make breaking that bad habit a very high priority!

Fasting for weight loss is rapidly growing in popularity due to its effectiveness in reversing diabetes and insulin resistance. Fitness enthusiasts have embraced the benefits of fasting, due to the increase in energy levels and rapid fat loss without compromising muscle mass. Top CEOs are even embracing fasting as a biohacking practice for its mental clarity and productivity benefits!

A study by scientists out of the University of Southern California showed that a 72-hour water fast effectively helps refresh the entire immune system. After around 24-hours the body is depleted of glucose and will simply begin to consume any damaged cells it finds for energy. Once you resume eating, your stem cells reengage to quickly replace the used cells.

When I first heard about this study on the radio one day while driving. I was fascinated and looked up the study to find out more prior to trying it for myself. During my first attempt at a 3-day water fast, I ended up falling a few hours short of the 72-hour window. I reached a point where I was a little shaky and decided to break my fast early. Three months later I tried again and was able to go for 84 hours! I now do a 72-hour water fast every three to four months to keep my immune system optimized.

Intermittent fasting has many health benefits. It has been proven to improve blood sugar control, boost brain function and even enhance longevity. In addition to promoting fat loss, fasting also improves blood pressure and cholesterol levels.

The biggest side effect from fasting is hunger. Contrary to what you may think, the hunger will begin to subside after the first couple of days as your body adjusts. Try drinking water, tea, or coffee when hunger strikes and try to stay busy. This will often make the hunger more tolerable or take your mind off the topic. Following the WFPB diet, where you eat a combination of high fiber, low carb foods, along with some good fat during your non-fasting mealtimes, will help. If hunger becomes too intolerable while attempting to fast, talk to your doctor about appetite suppression medications that may be an option for you. This can be helpful, especially in the beginning as your body adapts.

INTERMITTENT FASTING (IF)

"Fasting: More Powerful Than Any Drug on Earth" ~ **Movie, Directed by Doug Orchard**

Intermittent fasting is the term given to an eating pattern that cycles between periods of fasting and eating. It is also referred to as time restricted eating. Not only is it important to go for longer between eating (i.e. "fasting"), it is equally important that when you do eat, you consume the correct foods, and more importantly, avoid the wrong foods.

What are the "wrong" foods? All processed foods, sugar, and starches (bread, rice, potatoes, corn, peas). Your diet should consist primarily of whole, plant-based foods, mainly vegetables, and small portions of lean protein. Optimal snacks are calorie dense foods in small amounts, such as a small handful of nuts, a tablespoon of almond butter, or half an avocado. These will stop the hunger and satiate you for longer periods of time.

Fruit is allowed, but in very small amounts and only if your glucose is under control, since most fruit is high in sugar (remember we want to deplete all the glucose to "flip the switch" to fat burning for fuel). It is recommended that you limit fruit to berries and green apples at the start.

What about protein? As we discussed in an earlier chapter, contrary to popular belief your body needs far less protein than current culture believes and you can get all the protein you need simply from eating whole foods.

Don't like veggies? Roast them in the oven – they are delicious and so easy to make! Simply toss with some salt & olive oil and spread out on a pan. Place in 385°F oven for 20-25 minutes until they start to brown, or caramelize.

Vegetables are incredibly delicious roasted and I have had many skeptics change their mind after trying them. Brussel sprouts, cauliflower, broccoli, squash, onions, carrots, & sweet potatoes (in moderation) are all pleasing to the palate when roasted.

When using intermittent fasting, **what** food you eat is not as important as **when** you should eat. It is an effective way to lose weight, improve health and simplify your transition to a healthier lifestyle. Studies show that fasting can have a powerful effect on your body and brain, and may even help you live longer.

Fasting from time to time is actually more natural for the human body than eating 3-4 (or more) meals per day. Everyone naturally does intermittent fasts from time to time. If you have ever eaten dinner, then slept late and not eaten until lunch the next day, you've already done a 16+ hour fast. Some people instinctively eat this way - they simply do not feel hungry in the morning. Listen to your body and only eat when you are actually hungry. You do not have to eat breakfast immediately when you wake up!

How IF Effects the Body:

Several cellular and molecular changes happen in the body when you fast. The longer you go without eating, the more available glucose your body will use for energy. Once glucose is exhausted from the bloodstream, hormone levels change to make stored body fat the source of fuel for the body.

Studies show that people followed intermittent fasting for 24 weeks also lost 4-7% of their waist circumference. This indicates that they lost significant amounts of visceral fat, the harmful belly fat that builds up around the organs and can cause serious health problems.

However, keep in mind that the main reason IF works so effectively, is that it helps you eat fewer calories overall. If you binge and overeat during your meals you can easily reverse this benefit.

Health Benefits of IF:

In addition to ridding the body of fat, fasting has demonstrated many other health benefits.

- **Heart health:** Intermittent fasting may reduce blood sugar, triglycerides, LDL cholesterol, inflammation markers, and insulin resistance - all of which are risk factors for heart disease.

- **Cancer:** Animal studies show a reduction of cancer risk with intermittent fasting.

- **Brain health:** Intermittent fasting increases a brain hormone called BDNF and may aid the growth of new nerve cells. It may also protect against Alzheimer's disease.

- **Diabetes:** Risk of type 2 diabetes is lowered with intermittent fasting.

- **Insulin resistance:** Insulin levels can be reduced by 20-31% with intermittent fasting.

- **Anti-aging:** studies show that intermittent fasting even extends lifespan in rats.

- **Inflammation:** Studies show that intermittent fasting reduces inflammation markers, a key driver of many chronic diseases.

Eating healthy is fairly simple, but it can be incredibly hard to sustain. It takes some discipline to meal prep each week so that you have decent options available and are not tempted to eat fast food. Intermittent fasting is an attractive alternative since you do not have to plan, cook or clean up after meals, and it does not cost you anything. In fact, you can actually SAVE money, in addition to time, because you simply do not eat.

Different Styles of Fasting:

There are several different intermittent fasting styles. The three most popular methods are:

- **The 16:8 Method:** This is the most popular fasting method since it is the easiest and most sustainable. You simply reduce the consumption of all your daily food intake to 8 hours or less per day. This cycle can be repeated as frequently as you like — from just once or twice per week to every day, depending on the preference that works best for you. With this method you fast for at least 16 hours per day. While other diets often set strict rules and regulations, 16:8 intermittent fasting is easy to follow and can provide real results with minimal effort. It's generally considered less restrictive and more flexible than many other diet plans and can easily fit into just about any lifestyle. The most popular technique is to skip or eat breakfast later than usual and have dinner earlier than normal. Another option is to eat breakfast and lunch, then fast dinner and overnight. The warrior diet involves reducing the eating period to a four-hour period to promote an even deeper level of fat adaptation.

- **The 5:2 Method:** This is also a very popular method that involves eating normally 5 days a week, and eating only 500-600 calories on the other two, non-consecutive days. Bone broth or green smoothies are a good option with this plan. Many people find this way of eating to be easier to stick to than a traditional calorie-restricted diet. You can choose whichever two days of the week you prefer, as long as there is at least one non-fasting day in between them. One common way of planning the week is to fast on Mondays and Thursdays.

- **Eat-Stop-Eat:** With this method you fast for 24-hours, once or twice a week, then eat reasonably on the other days. The goal is to have a complete break from any calories for 24-hours at a time. An example would be to eat dinner then fast until dinner the following evening.

All three of these methods are effective, and can result in significant weight loss. I encourage you to try them all and see which one works best for you and what you currently have going on in your life. The longer periods without eating result in fewer calorie consumption overall and an effective lowering of stored glucose in the body. It may be difficult, especially the first time, as your body has to make adjustments. Each time you fast it will become easier.

Water, coffee, tea and other non-caloric beverages are allowed when fasting. Do not add sugar to your beverage, opt for stevia instead. While black coffee is highly recommended for optimal results, a very small amount of cream may be added if you absolutely must have some (no more than 1-2 teaspoons). Coffee can be particularly beneficial during a fast, because it can blunt hunger. You can also do a modified fast and have bone broth or a green smoothie as well.

Contrary to what cereal manufacturers want you to think, research shows breakfast is NOT the most important meal of the day. Forgoing breakfast, and thereby extending your overnight fasting state, is a far better option for weight loss and reduction of insulin sensitivity. It really is ok to skip breakfast!

It is important to take a quality multivitamin when fasting to ensure you replenish vitamins, minerals, and any electrolytes that may be diminished. However, keep in mind that some supplements, like fat-soluble vitamins, may work better when taken with meals.

You can continue to exercise while fasting without concern that you will lose muscle. Studies show that IF causes less muscle loss than regular calorie restriction diets. Muscle mass is actually preserved when fasting, due to the increase of growth hormone. Resistance training while fasting will even increase muscle mass! And, don't worry that fasting will slow your metabolism. Research shows that metabolism may actually increase while fasting up to 3 days as well.

While hunger is the main side effect with intermittent fasting, you should never feel bad. If you do start to feel weak, simply stop and eat. Most importantly, if you have a medical condition or are on medication you should consult with your doctor prior to trying any new program. This is particularly important if you are on any medication for blood sugar regulation.

Intermittent fasting is one of the best and simplest lifestyle changes that can improve your health. You do not have to go out and buy a bunch of special diet food or any special equipment. It is absolutely **FREE** - you simply do not eat. Again, the only thing you really have to lose is weight!

Bone Broth

"Good broth will resurrect the dead."
~ *South American Proverb*

Bone broth is recommended to use while fasting as it will supply vitamins, sodium, essential amino acids, and other minerals, all while helping to reduce hunger pangs.

Bone broth has been recognized for its many healing properties for centuries. Grandma actually knew what she was doing when she would make chicken soup anytime someone was sick!

When properly prepared, bone broth is a highly nutrient-dense food containing minerals, such as calcium and magnesium, and amino acids, that the body can easily absorb. Drinking broth each day can help to build muscle, reduce joint pain, fight infection, improve digestion, and detoxify. Bone broth is also full of collagen to make your skin look younger too!

Bone broth requires several hours of cooking time to obtain maximum nutrients and minerals into the broth. **Canned**

broth does not go through this process and therefore is missing many of the healing abilities we want to obtain with homemade broth.

Once cooled, a properly prepared broth will gel. The thicker the gel, the more nutrients it contains. If your broth is not jiggly when cooled then you probably added too much water or just did not let it cook long enough. The gel will dissolve when reheated and can be frozen for up to 6 months.

When preparing or prepping meals, save your vegetable scraps in a freezer bag to make your own delicious vegetable broth. For chicken bone broth, a shortcut I frequently use is to start with a fully cooked rotisserie chicken from the store. We will have some for dinner, then remove and portion or freeze the remaining meat, placing the skin, bones and carcass in the crockpot for our homemade broth.

The crockpot is the simplest way I have found to make a hearty bone broth. I simply add a couple celery stocks, onion, carrot, bay leaf, salt, garlic powder, black pepper, cover with water, and set to cook on low for 24 hours.

You can vary the broth recipe ingredients, changing the taste to the liking of your family. Freeze the broth in ice cube trays or single serving containers for convenience. Remember to leave at least 1 inch of extra space in the container for expansion; this is particularly important if freezing glass jars!

Green Smoothie Recipe

One option that has been very effective for many people is replacing breakfast (and/or lunch) with a healthy green smoothie. While they may not look tasty, they can actually be quite delicious. Here is a sample recipe of the one that I frequently make.

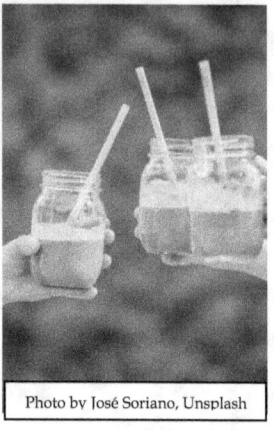

Photo by José Soriano, Unsplash

Equipment: VitaMix® blender (other blenders will work, but typically do not blend as smooth)

Add to your blender in this order:

- ½ cup water

- 1 scoop protein powder (if desired)

- 1 scoop chia seeds (this superfood will act as a thickener, optional)

- 1 scoop green powder

- Essential oils (I usually add 1-2 drops of ginger and dōTerra's OnGuard® Protective Blend)

- ¼ lemon, peel removed (any citrus will work, citrus helps remove the bitter flavor of the greens)

- 2-3 cucumber slices

- 1 stalk celery, cut into 1" pieces

- 2 cups tightly pack greens (I typically use a spinach/kale mixture

- Fresh parsley, to taste

- Fresh cilantro, to taste

- Stevia, to taste Photo by Jose Soriano, Unsplash

Blend well, then add ice to the desired consistency and enjoy! I prep and freeze most of the ingredients since I prefer a more frozen texture to my smoothie. Any leftovers can be refrigerated in a glass jar for the next day.

You can also use any veggies that you have. I sometimes use beets (and the green tops), any leafy greens I have in my fridge, squash, fresh mint, & more. A small amount of frozen berries, fruit, or avocado may also be added if the smoothie is not to be consumed during a fasting period.

Experiment with what you enjoy. I will sip on this during the morning and do NOT get hungry. In fact, I frequently have this for both breakfast and lunch!

Remember to drink plenty of water all day long and to take your supplements!

CHAPTER 12

KEEPING A FOOD DIARY

"What gets measured, gets managed." ~ **Peter Drucker**

A food diary is a fantastic way of keeping track of all the food that you consume. It will help you to be more conscious of how, what, and the amount you eat, and also help you stay accountable when setting and working towards your individual goals.

A food diary can also be helpful in identifying triggers of allergic or other reactions. It is a tool to help recognize and change habits since it tracks your intake in a very detailed manner.

Accountability really does help. Do you really know what you eat each day? Most people do not realize how much sugar they consume. Sugar comes hidden in many forms. As we discussed earlier, foods containing sugar are quickly converted to glucose by the body to constantly replenish your energy reserves, keeping your body in the fat storing state. This is opposite of where you want your body to be to lose weight.

You need to keep a food diary of every single thing you put in your mouth each day, especially in the beginning or if you plateau. If you eat a cup of Brussel sprouts, write it down; same goes for those two little M&Ms. You want to record each item consumed as soon as possible to avoid missing them.

Also jot down the quantity of each item. You can use measurements in volume, weight, or pieces. This helps you gauge how many servings you consumed. Remember to also note any extra toppings, such as butter, sauces, or condiments. Write down the time, where you were, and who you were with. You may want to also note what you were doing (watching TV, playing video games, etc.), as well as what kind of mood you were in while eating. Were you bored, sad, or joyful?

Each week, or even each evening, you can review what you have eaten and easily see where changes or adjustments need to be made. This discipline will help you, and your medical provider, identify bad habits early and see what modifications need to be made to maximize your efforts. It will also help you notice how frequently you are unconsciously snacking, or eating simply out of boredom or stress.

Keeping a diary of everything you consume does not have to be time-consuming or cumbersome and experts say most people will benefit from the effort. A food diary is one of the most effective tools to aid in changing your behavior.

There are numerous food tracking apps available, allowing you to immediately enter the info into your phone, at any time. You can include nutritional or other dietary information, organize and track foods by food group, and so on. This lets you monitor what, when, and how often you eat, as well as identify where any nutrition deficiencies may occur.

We have a free food diary template available on our website: I encourage you to download it and start keeping your food diary today!

CHAPTER 13

MEAL PLANNING AND PREP

"Those who think they have no time for healthy eating will sooner or later have to find time for illness."
~ Edward Stanley

If you find yourself asking each evening 'What should I/we have for dinner?', I would strongly encourage you to start planning your meals for the week in advance. The practice of advance preparation and portioning of meals is called meal prepping, and it can be a game changer, especially if you maintain a busy schedule. Prepping is also enormously helpful in helping you stay on track with the lifestyle changes you are making on your journey to optimal health.

Without a proper plan and some preparation, it is easy to fall off track and eat items that can threaten, or even derail, your success – especially when you get hungry!

I promise that meal planning will save you time, eliminate temptation, and help you make better food choices overall.

There really is not a right or wrong way to meal plan and prep, do whatever works best for you and fits with your schedule. Meal planning does not have to take a lot of time, and we even have a free template you can download on our website.

Meal planning and shopping

To get started look and make note of what food items you already have on hand. Next, make a template for the meals and any snacks you plan to have during the week, then create a shopping list from the plan of items needed. You want to ensure that you take a few moments to create your meal plan and go to the store to shop for food during a time when you are NOT hungry. If you shop while you are hungry you will be tempted to buy things that will undermine your efforts! For me, trying to shop while hungry just requires too much willpower.

When you go to the store, take your list and only purchase items on the list. Stick to the perimeter of the store since the heavily processed and junk food you want to avoid are usually located in the middle. I have also used the online shopping option offered by many stores near my home where you add what you need to your online order and just pick everything up at your scheduled pick-up time. If temptation is hard for you this may be a good option to try since some stores bring your order out to your car. I don't use this option as much as I used to, as I discovered I prefer to select my own produce. I also like getting fresh produce from my local Costco. I have found the pricing is lower, the produce is mostly organic, and the quality is good.

Another advantage to the online shopping option is that you do not have to even go into the store! This can come in handy when your schedule is particularly busy since you can do your "shopping" at anytime.

I generally go to the produce department first and fill my cart with a variety of wholesome vegetables and some berries. When I leave the produce area, I will head over to the frozen food aisle for fruits and vegetables.

The selection of frozen fruit and vegetables available nowadays is remarkable. Most are flash frozen at peak ripeness so they maintain their nutritional value and are more convenient. I appreciate having a wide variety of frozen fruits and vegetables year-round, when fresh options are not available or less than desirable. I was surprised to see that you can even buy avocado chunks for green smoothies!

Frozen vegetables and berries are definitely a time saver for me.

I like butternut squash, but do not necessarily like the labor involved to prepare butternut squash. Having the option to purchase it already peeled, cubed, and frozen makes preparing a roasted option or my favorite butternut squash soup much easier. The same thing goes for chopped onions and peppers. I can also use only the amount I need, which prevents waste. You can save both time and money using frozen veggies!

Outside of the produce and frozen veggie areas, the only other food items I frequently need are nuts, seeds, lentils, beans, spices, and coffee.

People think that it is expensive to eat a whole-foods, plant-based diet, but my total grocery bill has actually gone down. Reducing the amount of meat you consume will certainly lower your overall spend. You will also notice that when you avoid all of the pre-boxed, heavily processed options in the middle of the store, your total food bill is actually reduced. I find it quite ironic that the pre-processed items that are so bad for you are also the most expensive. Reduce your food budget, your waist line, and your consumption of artificial additives and preservatives by sticking to the perimeter of the store only.

Planning out your meals in advance and setting a little time aside for some prep work, will make it easier (and faster) to prepare your meals each day. Choosing in advance what you will eat each meal is not only more efficient, it is less stressful as well. How many times have you looked at whoever you are with and asked "what do you want for dinner?". The most popular answer is always "I don't know, what do you want?"! Do yourself a favor and download our meal planning template and shopping list today. Then start using it!

Using the template is quite easy and helps to eliminate waste from duplicate purchases. Simply look at what food you have on hand and jot down meals for the week that will use them. Then fill in the other meals with what you would like, noting any ingredients you need to complete the meals along the way.

If you have no idea what to make there are numerous websites that have countless ideas and recipes. Just search for "whole food plant based recipes". One of my favorites is pickuplimes.com. Other popular websites are makingthymeforhealth.com or forksoverknives.com. I challenge you to make their lasagna – it is absolutely delicious!

When you try a new recipe that you like, print it out or jot it down, along with any changes or notes you may need. Keep the recipes in an easy to find location to create your own collection of new dishes that you and your family enjoy. I have a three-ring binder full of the meals we enjoy most.

Keep in mind that in the beginning you want to stick with meals that include high fiber foods with low glycemic index scores. Meals that are higher in fat can be included time to time after you reach your initial weight goal.

You can also make changes to your old favorite recipes, making them compliant with your new way of eating. Noodles and pasta can be replaced with spaghetti squash or spiraled veggies, riced cauliflower makes a good substitution for white rice, butter can be replaced with unsweetened applesauce or avocado. Please do not think that you never get to have your old favorites again! Figure out a way to make substitutions to the recipe to and make them healthier instead.

Meal prep

Meal planning and prep has grown significantly in popularity over the past few years. It is not only healthy to plan and prep your food but also fulfilling to be in control of your time while you cook healthy and nutritious meals with less stress.

Prepping is the final step, coming after you have planned your meals for the week and shopped for the ingredients. It involves setting aside some time, to literally begin preparing, or prepping, the items you have for your upcoming weekly meals.

This can mean different things to different people, and it all comes down to what meals you have planned and what is the most helpful approach for your schedule and needs. Meal prep can involve making entire meals ahead, portioning them into individual containers, and then storing them in the fridge or freezer. It can also mean making a pot of beans, roasting some vegetables, or pre-chopping salad & smoothie ingredients.

I try to ensure I always have healthy snack options on hand and ready to go as well, so that I'm not tempted to stray and eat off my plan. For example, I will measure out a single serving of mixed nuts and place them in a small pill pouch on Sunday so I can just grab and go during the week. I also keep a pouch in my purse to have as a snack anytime I get hungry.

Meal prep ideas:

- Check your calendar – what do you have going on this week? What meals will you be eating out?

- Take a look in your pantry, fridge, and freezer – what do you already have that you want to use?

- Look up new recipe ideas online.

- Make your grocery list and then head to the store. Remember not to go when you are hungry!

- After shopping, sort food into make now or make later piles.

- Pre-wash, chop, slice, and peel any items to save time later in the week. You can store them in jars or Ziploc® bags.

- Store vegetable sticks upright in jars, adding an inch or so of water to keep them fresh and prevent dehydration.

- Premake salads in quart jars. Place the dressing on the bottom, then layer with ingredients, placing those with higher water content on the bottom. When you are ready to eat one, simply shake to mix and enjoy.

- Ensure that you stock your pantry with spices for additional flavor!

The overall purpose of meal prep is to save you time during the week, keep in mind however that not all food items can be prepped in advance or frozen. While prepared whole grains, soups, and chopped onions freeze well, salads do not. The life of refrigerated items and fresh produce should be taken into account when planning which meals to consume first as well.

The FDA has a PDF guideline available online showing the refrigeration and freezer time limits for many items. The container for storage can also impact the quality preservation of your prepped items. Storing items in individual sized containers is best, vacuum packing is even better to prevent freezer burn and oxidation. Also, keep in mind that liquids will expand when freezing so leave about an inch of extra room in your container to prevent breakage.

I recommend you start slow and prep for only 2-3 days in the beginning. Over time, you will learn what recipes tolerate prepping best and what meals you prefer made fully fresh.

Everyone can benefit from weekly meal planning. It is associated with a healthier diet and lower obesity rates. It is also one of the best weight loss "hacks" available since it helps to remove temptation when hunger strikes. With meal prepping you will have healthy snack options ready and available, so you do not even have to think about what to eat!

Save yourself time, frustration, and stress by beginning to meal plan and prep today.

CHAPTER 14

MINDSET MATTERS

"Thinking"
by Walter D Wintle

"If you think you are beaten, you are
If you think you dare not, you don't,
If you like to win, but you think you can't
It is almost certain you won't....

Life's battles don't always go
To the stronger or faster man,
But soon or late the man who wins
Is the man WHO THINKS HE CAN!"

Unity, 1905 edition, by Unity Tract Society, Unity School of Christianity

If you only take one piece of information from this entire book, I hope it is this – **mindset matters**! As the old adage goes "you are what you think!". If you want to achieve ANYTHING in life, mindset matters. Can you achieve a goal without the proper mindset? Of course, but I would argue that it makes the process much more difficult. So, why not help yourself by starting to cultivate a winning mindset from the start?

Your mindset and the way you think controls your entire life, how you perceive things, your emotions, and your actions. Your mindset is the life-long collection of experiences and beliefs that shape every decision you make, both conscious and unconscious. Mindset affects everything: how you think, what you feel, and what you do. It impacts how you see the world, and how you respond in any given situation. Your body is the outward result of what is going on inside the mind.

Most of the decisions you make each and every day are unconscious, guided by previous thoughts and experiences stored in your memory. The only way to reprogram the unconscious decisions made by your mind is by making a conscious decision to do so.

Consciously deciding to have a proper mindset when it comes to health and wellness is essential for success. Many times, people self-sabotage their efforts by simply thinking to themselves "it's not going to work" prior to even starting. I challenge you to retrain your brain starting today!

When you look at the most successful people, or anyone you want to emulate, one of the distinguishing factors they generally share is their positive mindset. They instinctively know and understand that they WILL achieve whatever goals they set for themselves. They can visualize the finish line from the beginning and then proceed to take the steps to make it happen!

If this does not occur naturally for you, there is a way to start promoting the practice of a positive mindset. Simply set aside a few minutes each day to focus on your goal. Close your eyes and visualize yourself at your optimal weight. What are you wearing? How do you look? What does it feel like? Now imagine yourself living in that future, because you will be!

Taking the time to visualize the feelings associated with achieving this goal is really important, so stay in that space for a moment and truly focus. Now start cultivating the belief that you can make this visualization a reality. Doing this simple visualization exercise each day will help you to stay on track to achieving this goal. We will cover more on this in the next chapter.

Another tip in changing your way of thinking is to say "I'm choosing to let go of excess weight", or "I'm giving my body permission to let go", instead of "I'm trying to lose weight".

Take a moment right now and say these phrases to yourself. Which one makes you feel better? You can hear and feel the difference! Mindset is crucial to achieving your personal goals.

You can manifest good, positive things in your life by simply thinking about, focusing on, and believing they can happen. Focus on the positive results of achieving your optimal weight – such as better health, a longer life, more enjoyment in everyday activities and the prevention of diabetes and heart disease. Focus on what you have instead of what you may have lost. Practice gratitude by writing down three things you are grateful for each day and surround yourself with positive people.

Also, celebrate your successes! Intentionally take time to appreciate the incremental goals you reach along the way. I broke my overall weight loss goal down into smaller portions. My first goal was 10 pounds. I took time to appreciate and celebrate when I reached this goal. I looked at myself in the mirror to truly see the changes. I made note of what articles of clothing were now loose. I celebrated each percentage point of reduction in my visceral fat level. You will gain additional encouragement when you take time to intentionally recognize that you successfully reached a goal. Then, you can simply set a new one.

Once I reached my original goal, I then made the increments smaller – only 5 pounds. I had already reached my goal, so each additional pound that I lost towards optimal was further success that I did not even consider obtainable at the onset. I successfully retrained my brain!

Goal setting does not come naturally for everyone. However, if you have a clear vision, set goals, focus & develop a plan, then act on that plan, I believe you will manifest amazing things in your life. Both my husband and I have successfully made several changes in my life over the last few years that prove this to be true.

I got serious about figuring out what it would take for me to successfully lose weight, reached (and exceeded) my goal weight in the process, resulting in a healthier, and happier, version of myself. I can honestly say that I am not the same person I was. I've effectively become a better version of myself; the way I saw myself in my mind's eye, the person I visualized. And, if I can do this, so can you!

CHAPTER 15

MEDITATION AND AFFIRMATIONS

"The goal of meditation isn't to control your thoughts, it's to stop letting them control you."

~ Anonymous

I will admit that when I began my journey just a short time ago, meditation was not a daily practice for me. I had never been one who enjoyed the practice of yoga or meditation. However, I came across a series of meditations specifically for weight loss during my research, and while I was skeptical, I decided to give them a try.

I knew that there was no way I was going to spend 30 minutes or more a day in meditation, but the meditations in this series were short, 10 minutes or less. Realizing how important mindset was for success and that meditation could help with mindset, I decided to listen to at least one meditation each day to see if it would make a difference.

The meditation series I tried is called *"The 21 Day Meditation for Weight Loss Challenge"* by **Jon Gabriel**. They cover many aspects of weight loss, such as absorbing nutrients, your ideal body, releasing stress, & digestive flow. There are numerous meditations such as these available online, and many are free. If you try one, but find you do not like the voice of the narrator or background music, simply try another. I would suggest you listen to a sample prior to any purchase and choose one that resonates with you, one you feel you would enjoy.

Personally, I was surprised at how much it helped to just spend 10 minutes a day listening and focusing on what my ideal body would look and feel like. After just a few days I noticed that it was easier for me to stay on track, I was not as hungry, and that I was losing weight faster! For the first time in my life, I was able to understand what a difference the practice of meditation could have for anyone, in any setting, in achieving a personal goal.

Remember how we covered how everything is made up of energy in an earlier chapter? The practice of meditation further drives this home. By simply taking the time to focus on what you would look and feel like in your ideal body, it creates the heart mind congruence that is essential for success in getting to that goal! The meditation aids the mindset.

If I had a day where I had to be at the office early, and did not have time to meditate at home, I would simply listen to the meditation recording in the car on my drive to or from work. **Warning**: never close your eyes and meditate while driving!

I discovered that even though I was not sitting with my eyes closed and "meditating", I was still benefitting from just listening! Just hearing the meditation recording helped to shift my mindset and give my body permission to let go of excess weight. The visualization you get from Jon's guided mediations is powerful, I encourage you to try them.

The benefits of meditation go far beyond mindset and stress reduction. Meditation has also been scientifically proven to control anxiety, lengthen attention span, and decrease blood pressure. You can also do it anywhere, at any time.

Affirmations

"Affirmations are like seed planted in soil. Poor soil, poor growth. Rich soil, abundant growth. The more you choose to think thoughts that make you feel good, the quicker the affirmations work." ~ **Louise Hay**

Incorporating positive affirmations into your daily routine is another practice that is proven effective for weight loss goals. Affirmations are brief phrases or sentences that are designed to encourage positive, happy feelings, thoughts, and attitudes. They can also be designed and written to specifically combat negative thoughts, feelings, and attitudes. This means that if you have an area that you struggle with, you can create an affirmation to aid in overcoming that specific struggle. An example of this would be the affirmation of "I love and accept my body" if you struggle with being ashamed or embarrassed with the way you look.

The key is that whatever affirmation you are using needs to resonate with you personally and align with your core values. Repeating an affirmation that you find on the internet but do not genuinely believe will not be as effective. It is also recommended that you say your affirmations daily, up to 3-5 times a day if needed. Post them on the mirror in the bathroom and say them to yourself each morning and every time you wash your hands!

Here are a few of the affirmations that I have used:

- I love and accept my body, appreciating the things it does for me.

- I freely release any guilt I have regarding food and eating.

- I am fully capable of reaching my ideal weight.

- My body absorbs nutrients from the healthy food I eat.

- I give myself, and my body, permission to let go of excess weight.

Saying specific and relevant affirmations to yourself in the mirror can motivate and encourage you to stay on track while simultaneously combating negative thoughts. One study even showed that daily affirmations encourage us to be more active and eat healthier. Practicing daily affirmations will help you develop a more positive mindset towards any goal you may have.

CHAPTER 16

CONTROLLING STRESS

*"The greatest weapon against stress is our ability to choose one thought over another." ~ **William James***

For most of us, stress is an everyday occurrence. Unfortunately, research reveals that stress can have a direct impact on the body including sleep disruption, headaches, chest pain, upset stomach, fatigue, and muscle tension or pain. Stress also affects our mood. When you are under stress, you may feel anxious, restless, overwhelmed, sad, depressed, or even angry.

Research shows that stress also has a direct impact on weight. Whether stress results in weight loss or weight gain will vary from person to person — and even situation to situation. In some cases, stress may lead to overeating; for others, stress may cause hunger to completely shut down, with no desire to eat whatsoever.

Chronic stress left uncontrolled can be dangerous, increasing your risk of heart attack & stoke, while weakening your immune system. Think of a time when you were really nervous and your heart was pounding. That is what stress can feel like in the body and mind.

The heart pounding is your brain sensing danger and switching you into what we call "fight or flight" mode. During this time the brain tells your cells to release adrenaline, which will increase your heart rate and blood pressure in preparation of helping you escape the perceived danger. At the same time, your body releases a surge of cortisol, which triggers your body to replenish the energy burst even though you have not actually used very many calories. The body will keep releasing cortisol for as long as the stress continues, and this can make you hungry - very hungry!

When you are in this situation your body will generally crave sweet, salty, and high-fat foods to stimulate the brain to release dopamine, the pleasure chemicals that activate the reward processing center of the brain. This soothing effect can become very addicting, but is completely opposite of where we want to be for optimal health. It is essential that you learn to control your stress level. The daily practice of meditation and affirmations will help in controlling and reducing stress levels.

Have fun

"We don't stop playing because we grow old; we grow old because we stop playing." ~ **George Bernard Shaw**

Having fun is one thing most of us do not intentionally plan for each week, however having fun matters. Scientific studies show that having fun gives your brain a chance to rest, thereby improving memory and concentration. Incorporating fun into your life improves your relationships, both personally and professionally, and is vital for combating stress.

I remember a time when one of my mentors asked me what I did for fun. I was surprised that I had to stop and think about it for a moment, only to realize that I had not really intentionally planned to do anything just for "fun" in quite a while. This was very eye-opening to me, but not to my mentor. He already knew that I was on a path to burnout and called me out on it with this simple question.

Now I make a conscious effort each week to schedule some fun time, such as time with my husband & family, a girl's night out, or lunch with friends. My husband and I have date night each Wednesday evening and we spend each Sunday afternoon with my daughter and her husband, having dinner or simply playing games.

Planning your week with intention, much like you preplan your meals, helps to ensure that the things that matter most actually get the time and attention they deserve. Not only does it provide you with necessary down time to recharge, it also helps to nurture your relationships. Chances are that if you do not preplan some fun time into your week, you will end up spending the entire week fighting various fires that pop up instead. Life will just get in the way.

Make having fun a priority by deliberately taking (and scheduling) time to enjoy the company of others, laugh with them, and simply have fun! Laughter and fun are good for you!

Self-care

"It's not selfish to love yourself, take care of yourself, and to make your happiness a priority. It's necessary." ~ **Mandy Hale**

Taking care of yourself is another vital piece to good stress management. In the hustle and bustle of the busy world in which we currently live, it is easy to let self-care get pushed to the wayside. This is especially true if you have young children or other caregiving responsibilities. Taking time for yourself is not selfish, on the contrary, it is a preemptive move to help prevent burnout. It is taking a few moments to practice some compassion for yourself to ensure that you can be your best for others.

Practicing self-care does not mean you have to go to a spa and get a massage either. It can be as simple as a relaxing soak in a hot tub after the kids are in bed (throw in some Epsom salt, baking soda, and essential oils). Self-care can also be reading a book or listening to music; for some people it's going to the gym. The importance is not the activity you choose, but rather that you intentionally schedule some downtime to refuel your needs.

It is unfortunate that we often do not take time to intentionally replenish our personal needs because we perceive this as being selfish. This is a false belief - quite the opposite is true! Not taking the time will lead to burnout. Self-care allows you to be a better, more authentic person. It also allows you to better care for others and helps to remind yourself that you are worthy. Because, my dear reader, you ARE worthy!

I encourage you to begin taking time each week to purposefully schedule time for fun and self-care in order to control your stress level. Living in a state of chronic stress, without downtime to refuel, puts your health at risk, elevates your cortisol and results in more visceral fat.

Now go schedule yourself a relaxing massage!

CHAPTER 17

DRINK YOUR WATER!

"Drinking water is like washing out your insides. The water will cleanse the system, fill you up, decrease your caloric load and improve the function of all your tissues."
~ Kevin R. Stone

Anytime you begin a new diet, exercise, or weight loss program, you will generally receive plenty of unsolicited advice from well-meaning friends, family, and even strangers. Out of these suggestions, one that is heard most frequently is "make sure you drink plenty of water". Turns out, this is actually a very sound piece of advice.

Staying properly hydrated is essential to life; every system of the body requires water to function. You can go for several days without eating, but only about 100 hours without water before your body will start shutting down. Continuing to go without water will eventually lead to death. The good news is that drinking water has been shown to aid with weight loss as well.

A 2016 study that measured participant hydration levels found that the less hydrated an individual, the more likely they were to have a higher body mass index (BMI). Inadequately hydrated individuals had a 60% higher chance of being obese over others that were suitably hydrated. Why the study did not prove that drinking water increased weight loss, it certainly showed a correlation between staying hydrated and lower body mass index. Additional studies have also shown drinking water to be beneficial for weight loss.

For the most part, we simply do not drink enough water. Instead, we opt for other fluids, like coffee or sodas, that can be dehydrating. One of the best habits you can cultivate is to drink a glass of water upon waking in the morning. Your body can become dehydrated overnight while you sleep. Drinking water first thing in the morning helps your kidneys efficiently flush toxins and kicks your metabolism into gear.

We also frequently confuse thirst as hunger. So, the next time you feel hungry, try drinking a glass of water first! Not only will it help with your hydration level, it will also make you feel fuller when you do eat.

Water has been shown to increase the resting energy expenditure of the body. This means you can burn more calories while resting just by drinking water. Cold water may even increase this further since the body must burn additional energy to heat up the water prior to digestion.

Benefits of drinking water & staying hydrated:

- Better digestion

- Improved cardiovascular health

- Less constipation

- Better joint lubrication

- Healthier skin

- Improved brain function

- Improved hormone production

- Helps the kidneys

- Better absorption of vitamins & minerals

- Efficient removal of waste

- Regulation of blood pressure

- Asthma & allergy reduction

- Improved physical performance

- Reduces hangover risk

The human body is approximately 60% water & water is the chief component in most body parts. So, exactly how much water should you drink each day? The general recommendation is one half to one ounce of water per pound of body weight. This means that if you weigh, say 150 pounds, you would need to consume 75-150 ounces of water each day. Another recommendation is to consume at least 8 ounces of water each hour you are awake. However, the best indicator of your hydration level is the color of your urine. When you are adequately hydrated the color of your urine should be light yellow to clear.

It is normal for your urine to be a brighter yellow shortly after taking your vitamins. A darker yellow or amber color is a reason for concern and an indicator of dehydration. It is easy to take a quick look in the toilet after you urinate. If the water is anything darker than a pale yellow you should probably drink some water!

Drinking adequate water each day to remain properly hydrated has numerous other health benefits. Did you know that headaches and high blood pressure can both be due to dehydration? I have repeatedly witnessed the elevated blood pressure of participants at health fairs reduce to normal levels just by drinking water!

Drinking water really does so much more than just quench your thirst. Staying properly hydrated also helps with digestion, reduces the risk of kidney stones, relieves constipation, improves brain function, and even helps prevent hangovers.

Water is needed by every cell of the body to get the oxygen, vitamins and nutrients they need. Your kidneys need water to help filter and flush toxins; water also aids the digestive system in the efficient removal of waste from the body. Water is critical for maintaining blood volume levels and brain tissue lubrication. Overall, proper hydration aids the entire body in working more efficiently. Now, go drink some water!

CHAPTER 18

SLEEP YOUR FAT AWAY

"The importance of sleep to healthy aging is often overlooked in the medical community, but it's becoming increasingly apparent that good sleep could be a new vital sign."
~ Dr. Robert Butler, National Institute on Aging

One area of your life that you may not realize has an impact on your health, specifically your waist line, is sleep. If you do not get enough sleep to properly restore and reset your body each evening it will actually store fat to compensate, specifically in the abdominal area. If you want to lose weight, or stay in a state of optimal health and wellness, be sure to get enough sleep.

According to the National Sleep Foundation, adults need at least 7 hours of sleep each night. One Gallup poll showed that over 40% of Americans are chronically sleep deprived, sleeping less than 7 hours a night. For teens it's even worse, with well over 90% of teens not getting their recommended 9 hours of sleep each night. Is it any wonder why Starbucks and energy drinks are so popular? Sleep deprivation has also been linked to insulin resistance, heart disease, and Type 2 diabetes.

What time you go to bed also has an impact on the quality of sleep you receive. Your body is genetically programed to automatically respond to light and darkness. In your brain, there is a tiny region behind the eye (above the optic chiasm), called the suprachiasmatic nucleus (SCN), that controls your circadian rhythm. This is the built-in 24-hour clock of your body, which naturally aligns with the 24-hour solar cycle of Earth.

When the sun goes down in the evening the SCN notices and sends a signal to your pineal gland, to start production of melatonin. This is the natural process that starts to make you drowsy, preparing you for sleep. In the morning, the reverse happens. The sun comes up, the morning light will signal your body to stop releasing melatonin, helping you to wake up.

During sleep your body naturally cycles through phases that last around 90-minutes of rapid eye movement (REM) sleep and non-REM sleep. Non-REM sleep is the deeper sleep period your body needs for recovery and recharging from energy exertion throughout the day. REM sleep is the period where your brain processes all the thoughts and memories that happened throughout the day and when you have the most vivid dreams.

Research shows that a higher percentage of deep non-REM sleep occurs during the first half of the night, between 10:00 pm and 3:00 am, whereas REM sleep is higher in the early morning hours, 2:00 am to 7:00 am. When you understand this, you can see why people who stay up later do not awaken as refreshed as those who go to bed earlier, even with the same number of hours slept. Their body simply has not received as much of the non-REM deep sleep to fully recover.

Workers with night shifts have a higher probability of being overweight than coworkers who have day shifts as well. If you do have to work nights, strive to get at least 7 hours of sleep, preferably in a dark and quiet environment. Use a white noise machine to drown outside noise and aid sleep quality.

Another correlation between lack of sleep and weight gain has to do with two not so well-known hormones, leptin and ghrelin, both of which deal with hunger and appetite.

Only discovered in 1994, leptin is a hormone that helps to regulate your energy levels by inhibiting hunger. Levels are increased when sleeping, since your body needs less energy then. Being sleep deprived decreases leptin production so your brain thinks that you need to eat, even when it is not necessary. Additional research shows that leptin plays a role in other areas, including brain function, bone formation, immunity, sexual development, and fertility.

Ghrelin is the hormone produced in the stomach that makes you feel hungry. In the body, ghrelin works in the opposite way of leptin, production of ghrelin is decreased while sleeping. Not getting enough sleep makes your body produce more ghrelin, thereby making you feel hungry, in addition to grouchy from being sleep deprived!

Not getting sufficient sleep to recharge each evening will slow down your metabolism and result in elevated hunger levels from these two hormones not being properly reset each evening. Your brain reasons that you need additional energy and will continue in a fat storing mode until you are fully rested.

Sleep disorders also cause sleep interruption and deprivation, effecting over 25% of U.S. adults. Left unreported and undiagnosed, sleep disorders can even be dangerous. Sleep apnea, a condition where normal breathing is interrupted during sleep, has been linked to heart disease, stroke, hypertension, and cognitive impairment. Snoring can be another indicator that you are not getting quality sleep. Talk to your doctor about any concerns you may have regarding your sleep, if it takes you more than 30 minutes to fall asleep, you are not waking up feeling rested, or if you have daytime fatigue.

Signs that you're not getting enough sleep:

- Not feeling well rested upon waking after spending more than 7 hours asleep

- Feeling sleepy during the day

- Falling asleep within 5 minutes when having an opportunity to nap

- Falling asleep unexpectedly or at inappropriate times during the day

- Needing to use stimulants to stay awake during the day

- Others report you snore, snort, gasp, or make choking sounds while you sleep

- Others notice you stop breathing for short periods

- Frequently waking up during the night with difficulty falling back to sleep

- Difficulty in getting moving when you first wake up

- Sudden jerking of the arms or legs during sleep

If you have trouble falling asleep there are several things you can try. I tend to wake up fairly easy from outside noise so I use a white noise machine. When it is on, all outside noises are masked and it helps to lull me into sleep quickly. I even have a white noise app on my phone and iPad that I use when traveling.

While prescriptions for sleeping pills are widely available, there are certain supplements available that may help you fall asleep just as well. Melatonin can help you fall asleep and is especially helpful when you need to adjust to a new time zone. Magnesium, GABA, and 5-HTP have also been shown to help with sleep. I personally take magnesium, zinc, and GABA each evening.

Caffeine is a stimulant that can keep you from falling asleep. If you are caffeine sensitive, limit or eliminate caffeine from your diet 4-6 hours prior to bedtime. Although alcohol is frequently used as a sleep aid, and may make you feel drowsy, it negatively impacts your quality of sleep by reducing REM sleep. For some, exercising in the hours just before bed can inhibit sleep as well. Exercise in the morning hours is a better option.

Tips for falling asleep:

- Turn off all electronics at least an hour before bed

- Use a white noise machine

- Take a warm, relaxing bath before bed. Use Epsom salts, baking soda, & essential oils to pamper yourself.

- Listen to some soothing music or try reading

- Diffuse essential oils

- Go to bed at the same time each night

- Turn down the thermostat. You sleep better in a cool environment.

- Make your bedroom a comfortable, quiet, & dark sanctuary for sleep and sex only. No working in bed!

- Avoid caffeine in the afternoons since it can stay in your system 4-6 hours

- Stop eating at least 3 hours before bedtime

- Go out in the sun every day. Sunshine regulates your internal clock and helps you stay alert.

- Turn down the lights at sunset. Darkness is the body's cue to prepare for sleep.

Stop any exercise and do not eat anything for at least three hours before you go to bed. Try going to bed earlier if you feel tired during the day. Track your sleep for a week to ensure you are actually sleeping at least seven hours each night. I prefer to get up by six o'clock each morning, so I try and go to bed around ten each evening. If I have to get up earlier, I will adjust my schedule accordingly, and go to bed earlier. I may stay up a little later on the weekends since I know I can sleep in the next morning. Try and keep your schedule as consistent as possible for best results. Night, night!

CHAPTER 19

GET MOVING

"To enjoy the glow of good health, you must exercise."
~ Gene Tunney

Yes, maybe when you were a teenager you could eat whatever you wanted and still stay thin. Let's be honest though, more than likely you were much more active during those years too. As we age, our bodies change and our metabolism slows. We must mature and change our attitude towards both movement and the way we eat.

Contrary to what our culture would have you believe; exercise is absolutely NOT the best or most efficient way to burn fat. The truth is, fitness begins at the table, and no amount of cardio or crunches can sculpt a sleek physique if you maintain an unhealthy diet. It is simply impossible to exercise your way out of a bad diet! Cutting the calories to begin with is way easier.

So, what about exercise? How should it fit into your overall program? Unless you are an extreme athlete, exercise rarely has a significant impact on the overall quantity of fat burned for energy. This is because exercise will trigger your body to replenish used energy and actually increase hunger. For this reason, we usually recommend you not begin an exercise program during the first few weeks of starting any type of program designed to reduce weight. Of course, you may continue to exercise if you already have regular exercise as a part of your normal schedule. We have just found it far easier to wait until your body is recovered from sugar withdrawal, and adjusted to your new way of eating and fasting, to incorporate exercise and movement into your daily routine.

Please understand, we are **NOT** saying that exercise is not important, quite the contrary, exercise is one of the most important factors in improving health, especially for longevity. Exercise is the best thing you can do to strengthen your heart and lungs, lower cholesterol, improve mood, and even sleep better.

Another benefit of exercise is that it helps to optimize insulin and leptin receptor sensitivity, thereby normalizing glucose, insulin, and leptin levels. Not only are these essential for weight loss but also prevention of disease.

Before starting any exercise program, it is advisable to discuss it with your personal physician. They can make recommendations for what may be appropriate for you and what movements, if any, should be avoided.

What is the best and most efficient type of exercise? According to research, short, sprint recovery style workouts, even ten minutes or less, and walking 7,000-10,000 steps per day. Why sprint-recovery? Obviously for time, but also for numerous other health benefits, including improved cardiovascular health, boosted metabolism, and overall muscle building & conditioning.

Despite widespread belief, more is not better for your health when it comes to exercise, making sprint recovery workouts the most beneficial style of exercise for heart patients.

"Darwin was wrong about one thing. It's not survival of the fittest, but survival of the moderately fit ... We weren't born to run. We were born to walk, and we need to be walking more ... you need to be moving your body more than sitting

- every chance you get, move!" – **TED Talk by Dr. James O'Keefe, research cardiologist and former elite athlete.**

Multiple studies have shown that a ten-minute sprint recovery style workout is as, or even more, effective to an hour or more on the treadmill. During the "sprint" part of the workout, a duration of 20-30 seconds, you give the exercise all that you have, working your muscles as hard as you can. This has the advantage of kick-starting your metabolism, causing your body to continue burning calories long after you have finished. And, who doesn't like being more efficient? I certainly do. With my crazy schedule it is difficult for me to find a two-hour block of time to go to a gym, however I can always squeeze in 10-15 minutes. Plus, I can do this style of exercise anywhere, at any time, since no special equipment is required.

Another benefit is that I do not even need to change clothes since I'm not sweating much, like you can from normal workout routines. I generally do my routine sometime over the lunch hour, which is best for me since I fast lunch most days. I start with 1-2 minutes of stretching or walking on the treadmill to warm up, then 20-30 seconds of sprint exercise, followed by two minutes of passive recovery. Then I repeat using a different exercise and passive recovery, and repeat again. I vary the movements to ensure I get all muscle groups during the week.

Sample routine:

- **30 seconds** squats (Begin with legs hip width apart and arms down by your sides. Lower your body down into a sitting position, the straighten your legs to stand. Repeat quickly for the full 30 seconds.)

- **2 minutes** of gentle knee to hands (Start in a natural standing position with feet hip width apart. Lift up right knee and touch to your right palm, gently alternate to the other side, back and forth for the time period.)

- **30 seconds** of jumping jacks (Stand with feet together and legs slightly bent, arms at your side. Jump while raising arms above head and spreading legs apart. Jump back to starting position and repeat.)

- **2 minutes** of gentle, open palm twists (With slightly bent knees and arms extended out, turn palms of hands up towards the sky. Gently twist entire torso and swing arms left to right, while keeping feet in place.)

- **30 seconds** of climbing the wall (Start in upright standing position, with arms up in front, bent, with palms facing out. Jog in place while moving opposite arm up towards the sky, like you're climbing a wall.)

- **2 minutes** of gentle stretch and reach (With arms above head, inhale while reaching as far back as you can stretching your core, then exhale while stretching forward letting your fingertips touch the ground. Repeat.)

Total time: 7.5 minutes

Remember, for best results you need to give it your all during the shorter sprint portion! You should be out of breath when you are done, which you will be able to recover from during the longer passive recovery stage. Following these 2 minutes of warmup, and 3 sprint recovery phases, I simply do a 2-5-minute walk to cool down again.

There are numerous free videos and programs for this exercise style available online to choose from if you need help getting started. Just search for "high intensity interval training". One of my favorites is a series by Meredith Shirk called "One and Done". I must give her credit for convincing me through the simplicity in her videos that I could incorporate a short sprint-recovery workout into my crazy schedule and still get amazing results. She even covers modifications for some movements, in case you have any limited mobility or injuries.

Walking is another underrated activity that has a wonderful impact on health. Since walking is a lower impact activity it can be a better option for some, especially if you have knee or back pain. Walking outside is better, since being out in nature has shown to reduce stress and anxiety. You can get the same results by mimicking the sprint-recovery routine above. After an initial warm up, walk at a faster pace or on an incline to elevate your heart rate, followed by a slower pace for recovery, then repeat. This fluctuation of raising and lowering the heart rate has the maximum fat burning effects.

Exercise can be fun, quick, and easy! If you find one type of exercise boring, just find something different to do. It also helps to have someone else to workout with, especially in the beginning. You can help hold each other accountable to get your movement minutes in each day and encourage each other to do more.

Incorporating movement into your daily routine has many positive health benefits. Although exercise alone is not a good weight management strategy, it is an essential piece of the puzzle for optimal health and longevity. And, it is never too late to start either. Seniors who start a movement routine have some of the best benefits, including reduced disease risk, increase in cardiovascular strength, improved flexibility, and fall prevention.

I challenge you to start incorporating at least 10-15 minutes of simple exercise and movement into your day. Vary your movements to include all muscle groups over the week. Start out with a goal of just 3 days a week, then work up to 60 minutes total a week - that's less than 10 minutes a day! You will be surprised how quickly you build strength, feel better, and start enjoying this part of your day.

Remember to check with your personal doctor before starting any new exercise program, especially if you have not exercised for a long time, have health issues, heart disease, diabetes, or any other concerns.

CHAPTER 20

PUTTING IT ALL TOGETHER

"I learned a few years ago that balance is the key to a happy and successful life, and a huge part of achieving that balance is to instill rituals into your everyday life - a nutritious balanced diet, daily exercise, time for yourself through meditation, reading, journaling, yoga, daily reflection, and setting goals." ~ Gretchen Bleiler

"A goal without a plan is just a wish."
~ Antoine de Saint-Exupéry

As you can see, when it comes to sustainable weight loss, there are many pieces involved to solve the puzzle. The way the pieces fit together is different for each individual as well. It really is a trial and error task to figure out the solution to the plan that is effective for you!

The first step is to make up your mind that you are determined to see this through and work with your personal medical provider to make a plan and obtain baseline testing. Next, learn what foods to eat and avoid to deplete your body of glucose and successfully switch to burning fat for fuel. Then train yourself to plan out your meals, make out your shopping list and purchase only the items needed, then prep in advance for fast and easy meal options during the week. During meals, slow down and consciously enjoy your meal; intentionally take time to fellowship with those around you and chew longer.

Purposefully focus on your mindset each day; take your recommended supplements and always drink plenty of water. Learn to successfully control your stress and strive to obtain adequate sleep each evening.

In this book, we introduced intermittent fasting and showed how it can be a very powerful ally on your journey, both in overall weight loss and in helping to get past a plateau. We have provided examples of different meditation styles and affirmations, explaining how they can play a significant role as well.

I have given you a starting point for many of the pieces that I personally found essential. Now it is your responsibility to learn more about each piece that resonates with you, as you implement the related actions into your personal solution. I encourage each of you to persist, as I had to do, so that you too can reach, and even surpass, your personal optimal health and weight goal.

Remember - life happens and will often get in the way. You will cheat, and feel like you failed from time to time, but it is not the end of the world. Practice compassion - forgive yourself and move on, simply starting again.

Stumbling does not mean that you failed, so do not ever use it as an excuse to stop. **Never give up on yourself or your goal!** It is also important to appreciate that being "skinny" by itself will not necessarily make you happy; happiness is a choice. I so hope that you will choose to be happy!

Let your personal journey to optimal health begin!

More information, additional tools, and resources can be found on our website: **bigfatpuzzle.com**.

www.ingramcontent.com/pod-product-compliance
Lightning Source LLC
Chambersburg PA
CBHW070833310526
45788CB00017B/560